SuperPowers of the Family Kitchen

From the Author of
SuperPowers, A Busy Woman's Guide to Health and Happiness

SUPER POWERS

of the

Family

Kitchen

Adita Yrizarry-Lang

Learn how to feed kids to be SuperPower STRONG!

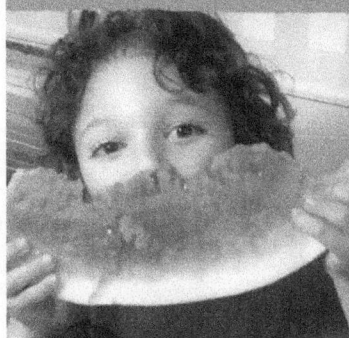

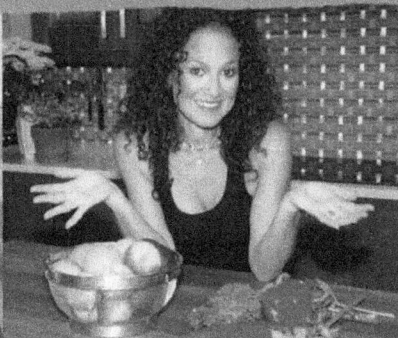

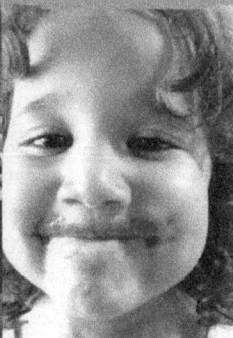

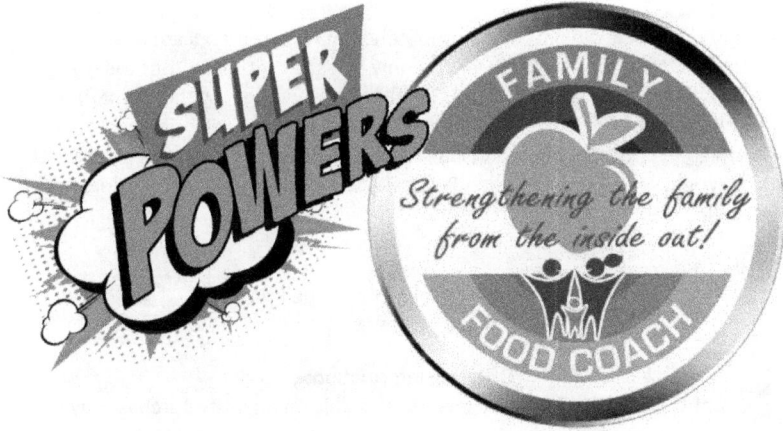

"Empower Yourself with Knowledge!" and maximize the benefits from everything that you feed yourself and your family. Food selection should enhance your family's Immune System, Health, and overall Mental Wellness and Development. Adita will guide you through all of the confusion and teach you the fundamentals of creating just the right food plan for your family's needs. Understand the basis of health through proper food selection; create yummy food plans that enhance brain development and growth; understand food challenges that can affect self-esteem and health; and change your family's view on food for the better! Food planning should not be a chore, and creating the right plan with the foundation for a healthy pallet should come with ease, providing benefits for years to come.

Published by SuperPower Blue Print

Ordering Information:
Quantity sales - Special discounts are available on quantity purchases by corporations, associations, and others. For details, contact info@AditaLang.com
Orders by U.S. trade bookstores and wholesalers. Please contact info@AditaLang.com

Paperback ISBN: 978-1-7325351-2-1

Ebook ISBN: 978-1-7325351-3-8

Library of Congress Control Number:2019907718

Cover Illustration Copyright © 2019
Cover design by JAS Designs
Book design and production by Adita Yrizarry-Lang

Disclaimer

The information is this learning work is in no way intended as medical advice or as a substitute for medical counseling. This publication contains the opinions and ideas of its author. It is intended to provide helpful and informative material on the subjects addressed in the publication. It is sold with the understanding that the author and publisher are not engaged in rendering medical, health, psychological or any other kind of personal professional services in the book. If the reader requires personal medical, health or other assistance or advice, a competent professional should be consulted. The author and publisher specifically disclaim all responsibility for any liability or loss, personal or otherwise, that is incurred as a consequence, directly or indirectly, of the use and application of the contents of this book. Before starting a weight loss plan, a new eating program or beginning or modifying an exercise program, check with your physician to make sure that the changes are right for you.

TABLE OF CONTENTS

Stay Connected:

http://www.twitter.com/AditaLang

www.facebook.com/AditaLangWellness

http://www.linkedin.com/in/AditaLang

http://www.youtube.com/Aditalang

http://www.pinterest.com/AditaLang

http://www.instagram.com/AditaLang

For more information on classes and speaking engagements by Adita, check out http://www.AditaLang.com

About the Author

Adita Yrizarry-Lang is Nash and Mila's mom. She is also a SuperPower aficionado, author of *SuperPowers, A Busy Woman's Guide to Health and Happiness*, and a speaker. Her "Journey" started as a certified fitness instructor 30+ years ago. Since her initial beginnings, she expanded her endeavors to specialize, from a biomechanics and resistance training expert to nutritional guru, mind-body serenity coach to advocate for family health and nutrition. Adita holds a BS in Holistic Nutrition, is a Lv3 Holistic Lifestyle Coach through the Chek Institute, and has been accredited by several respected organizations, including NASM, ACE, AFAA, and the University of Miami. She is a faculty member for The International Sports Conditioning Association, Wellness Director for Fierce4 Fitness, and the developer of the online course Nutritional Brilliance. She has trained thousands of fitness professionals' worldwide and often speaks at schools, Fortune 500 companies, and private organizations on the benefits of quality foods, longevity, and amazing health.

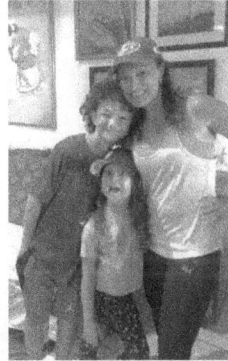

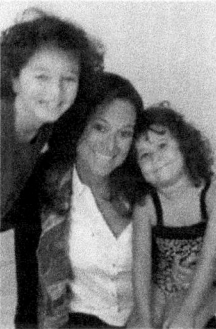

Adita's mission now...Inspire families to live life with their true potential in the forefront. Share the easiest ways of incorporating healthy rituals so that they become lifelong habits. And through social media, blog posts, and video she wants to bring out the trials and tribulations of life and offer solutions that can be easily incorporated into one's day to make SuperPowers shine and life thrive on, better than ever!

SuperPowers of the Family Kitchen
Introduction

As parents we pride ourselves in our kids, we want them to strive for success and enjoy the endless adventures in front of them. We try to give them the very best and we want them to grow up smart, strong, and full of energy (OK, maybe not too much energy). We read a few things here and there, listen to our friends and family, and hope that we are giving them the right foods, but with time against us on a day-to-day basis we tend to settle, leaving some of those choices to challenge the health of our family for years to come. You are growing an adult from scratch with every bite that you feed a child. Every food choice made is creating the foundation of health for your children that will actually affect them through adulthood.

This book is designed to teach you about Food Based Nutrition, what I like to call "the Nutraterian Approach". In other words, I want you to learn about healthy FOODS, about eating for nutrition and eliminating any advice towards supplementation or synthetically derived food sources. You have the power to enhance your family's lifestyle by helping them make better choices, eat healthier, and by creating their pallet of flavors that enhances their health for a lifetime!

1

Many families struggle with everything from hyperactivity to weight loss, then there are those who don't understand the consequences of their choices, who are challenged with low energy, memory fog or a low immune system without even realizing it. Food is very powerful and the right choices can enhance someone's day-to-day. As the head of your household you have the power to change and alter taste buds in favor of health and vitality. It is never too late to turn it all around. Now, granted, for some of you this change may take more time than you had thought, but your dedication and creativity will be much more valuable than anything modern medicine can serve up.

Knowledge and encouragement will serve your family the very best of all. Your motivation and enthusiasm can impact someone's life in an amazing way, and we all realize that food can expedite or slow down this process. It is important to recognize that every individual has their own unique set of nutritional needs, so your job is to guide your family in the right direction, assist them, and, if needed, find a licensed professional who can customize a food plan, prescribe supplementation or simply provide you the right foundation for the specific health needs of the family.

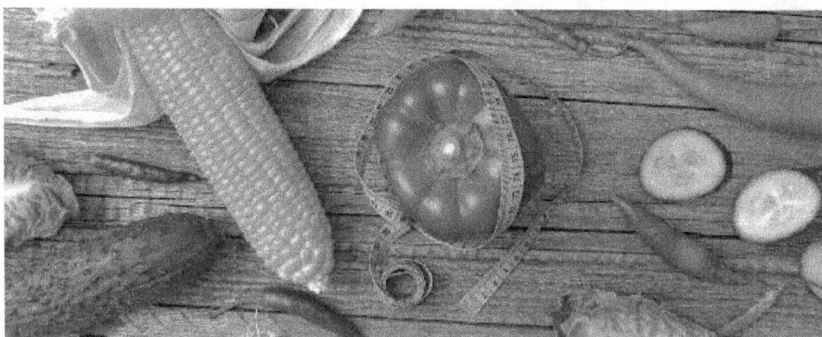

SuperPowers of the Family Kitchen was created to teach you everything you need to know about how to feed your family right. We are all very different in how we metabolize food, digest food, lose weight, etc. The knowledge you gain as you read this book is designed to target those with good general health. Many times we deal with family members who have medical issues, take medications or just don't want to change; when we reach some of these walls, it's time to call in reinforcements. I like to have a strong network of professionals that can help me fill in the gaps when needed. The following is a list of various nutritional professionals; it is important to understand the basis of each in order to make the right choices for your family's needs.

Registered Dietician - The American Dietetic Association defines a Registered Dietitian (RD) as "a food and nutrition expert who has met the minimum academic and professional requirements to qualify for the credential 'RD'." These individuals can prescribe nutritional supplements and specific food plans that are created in conjunction with medical intervention.

Nutritionist - A nutritionist is commonly defined as a person who advises people on dietary matters relating to health, wellbeing and optimal nutrition. Unfortunately, there is no legal definition for nutritionists so their educational level can vary from a simple continuing education course all the way up to a master's degree in chemistry. When working with nutritionists, investigate their background to fully understand their level of education and expertise.

Nutritional Counselor - Again, without legal definition, this person may or may not have the level of education that is needed to work with you and your family. Typically a nutritional counselor cannot prescribe supplements, but they act as an educator for you to decide what would work best for you and the family—more as a nutritional consultant.

Holistic Nutritionist - Holistic healing is a facet of alternative medicine that focuses on healing the body as a whole in order to cure illness and disease—mind, body, and spirit. Traditional nutrition looks at a specific problem, such as weight loss. They then work on a calorie count as opposed to the quality of the food choices and the reasons behind the weight gain in the first place. Holistic practitioners rely on well-balanced food plans of natural ingredients and look for the quality of and effects of foods more so than their caloric values.

Homeopath - This is one who works on curing the body as a whole with the use of herbs and specialized treatments that mimic the illness in order to assist the body in combating the problem. According to Wikipedia, a 2005 survey revealed that 100,000 physicians worldwide utilize homeopathy with the majority of their patients.

Naturopathic Doctor (ND or NMD) - This is a complementary and alternative medicine that utilizes the body's natural ability to heal and maintain health. Traditional naturopathy uses herbs and food as opposed to surgery and synthetic medicines. They are legally protected in several US states and can use traditional diagnostic tests, such as blood tests and imaging, in order to identify any health issues.

As you read this book some things may seem casual and others may seem technical, don't let it distract you, I realize your time is precious but all of this will come together in a nice package as you read through it all. At the end, all of the food and nutrition stuff will feel like a pretty easy mastery, I promise!

"The last birthday party we went to a mom gave my son a huge piece of cake. I, of course, cringed but within seconds my son had taken a few bites and then told me he was done. He said 'mom this is way too sweet, do I have to eat it?', halleluiah a low sugar pallet can taste the sweetness super quick!!"

Notes, Stuff to Remember, Things to Buy, etc.

Nutrition 101

Nutrition is the process of nourishing the human body by the assimilation of food and utilizing its properties (i.e. nutrients) for the growth and replacement of tissue. In addition, it is the science of understanding food, its properties, and its effects on the human body and mind. Studies show that people committed to an exercise program, tend to eat well and are more mentally alert. With life's many challenges, stress can wreak havoc on the internal system. Exercise helps to defuse that stress, but inadequate nutrition can deplete the immune system and exacerbate undetected health issues, making nutrition an integral part of health.

OK, here is where some of the science kicks in, work with me people. This will all fit together in a nice nutritional package designed for YOU and the members of your family at the end, you got this!

Nutritional Components

The human body requires six nutrient components in order to assure normal growth and function. These components are the nutritional precursor that enhances the human body by providing energy, creating building material, repairing and maintaining tissue, promoting and sustaining growth, and regulating and assisting in every function and process of the body. These nutritional components are broken down into the following categories: Carbohydrates, Proteins, Fats, Vitamins, Minerals, and Water. Below is a very simplified breakdown to give you a general understanding of the most common nutritional components. Keep in mind that there are several additional classifications for vitamins and minerals and these can be studied in specialized nutritional courses or can be discussed further through a licensed practitioner.

Carbohydrates

They are a primary source for energy and provide 4 calories per gram. Glucose is the sugar that is produced by carbohydrates and it is a main source of energy in both the mind and body. Carbohydrates are broken down into two categories:

- *Simple* – These carbohydrates are easily digested, in other words they provide immediate energy but for a very short period of time and are not the best source of energy for prolonged exercise and activity. These include sugar, white flour, processed cereals, cookies, etc. Most manufactured or processed foods would fall under this category. They metabolize as a sugar and are stored as fat if not utilized for immediate energy. They also include corn syrup and high fructose corn syrup, which many manufactures use as an inexpensive form of sugar although it has been linked to obesity, high cholesterol, and many other diseases.

- *Complex* – This form of carbohydrates requires a bit more in the digestive process, which will give you a longer steady stream of immediate energy due to its vitamin and fiber content. These include fruits and vegetables, grains and unprocessed cereals. They are comprised of dietary fiber, which assists in the elimination of toxins in the body and provides an excellent source of energy for both the mind and the body. Complex carbohydrates provide optimal energy and nutrients when they are minimally processed or cooked below 105 degrees. Combined with quality fat and proteins, complex carbohydrates can give sustained energy for a long period of time.

Proteins

These take much longer to digest. I call these the things that provide "cruise control" to your energy centers yet provide 4 calories per gram. They include chicken, fish, meat, eggs, grains, leafy greens, seeds, and nuts. Protein is a source of energy that comes with a delay in digestion, which does not make it a good source for immediate energy. On the other hand, when it is combined with complex carbohydrates (primarily fruits and vegetables), it slowly releases the complex carbohydrates into the system, allowing the body to maintain its energy for a longer period of time.

Proteins are considered the building blocks of the body; every cell in the human body contains protein, and they help to build and repair cells as well as muscle tissue. At least 10,000 different proteins make you what you are with your unique framework of strength, health, and overall longevity.

Proteins are made up of hundreds of thousands of smaller units called amino acids, which are attached to one another in long chains. There are 20 different types of amino acids that can be combined to make a protein. The sequence of amino acids determines each protein's unique 3-dimensional structure and its specific function.

Our bodies make amino acids in two different ways: either from scratch or by modifying protein sources. A few amino acids (known as the *essential* amino acids) must come from food.

- Animal sources of protein tend to deliver a complete amino acid chain.
- Other protein sources, such as fruits, vegetables, grains, and some nuts and seeds, lack one or more essential amino acids but they can be acquired by combining foods in order to complete the chain (beans and rice or garbanzos and tahini for hummus).

Vegetarians need to be aware of this. People who don't eat meat, fish, poultry or eggs need to eat a variety of protein-containing foods each day in order to get all the amino acids needed to make a complete protein.

Amino acids are classified into three groups:

Essential   Nonessential   Conditional

Essential amino acids cannot be made by the body and must be supplied by food. They do not need to be eaten at one meal. The balance over the whole day is more important.

Non-essential amino acids are made by the body from essential amino acids or in the normal breakdown of proteins.

Conditional amino acids are needed in times of illness and stress.

Some children will eat animal products, others won't, but as a parent it is your job to make sure that every meal and snack incorporates a sufficient amount of protein to help regulate energy and provide a good foundation for proper growth.

Several health authorities and schools come up with guidelines in regards to specifically "how much" protein every age group needs. It can become a bit overwhelming, but for our purposes it is important to recognize that a growing body needs protein for proper growth and development.

So How Much Protein Do We Need? Here's the thing; we each metabolize foods in a very unique manner and we each have a different need for protein in our day-to-day food plan. Initially, the easiest way to distribute protein portions for the average person is to start with a protein base of 40% of the meal or snack. From here you start to see how "hungry" you are before your next meal or snack. In other words, if you come to your next meal or snack and you are famished, you probably didn't have enough protein in the meal before. If you really pay attention to your hunger and the hunger of your family, you will come to see how each person's protein needs vary. From there the following will give you some basic examples that will help modify the proportion of protein needed per meal and/or snack:

Daily Activity Level – A lot of exercise would require more protein for muscular repair.

Daily Food Planning – If there is ample time between meals, you would increase your protein and fat proportion so that the calories would last longer in your system. For your kids, you have to plan breakfast with the knowledge of them having/not having a snack and what time lunch is set at during school days. When they are at home, you have more flexibility, but when they are at school, you have to plan your food proportions with the time between meals that the school imposes.

For High Stress or Illness – High quality, nutritionally dense proteins would need to be added.

Fats

These have had a "bad rap" throughout the years. They are comprised of 9 calories per gram and are basically simple to understand. For your purposes, there are two forms of fat—good and bad. The right fat can help to provide energy to the body; as with protein it takes longer to digest but can assist in a long-duration activity. In addition, if combined correctly, fats can slow down the spike of both sugar and caffeine, assisting our energy receptors and maintaining energy for a longer period of time.

Bad Fat (the following information is retrieved from The Mayo Clinic.org):

- *Saturated fat* - This is a type of fat that comes mainly from animal sources, it can be cut off of animal proteins such as meat, is a thicker denser substance as in butter or lard, and is also found in full-fat dairy products. Saturated fat raises total blood cholesterol levels and low-density lipoprotein (LDL) cholesterol levels, which can increase your risk of cardiovascular disease. Saturated fat may also increase your risk of type 2 diabetes. It also happens to be the place where all toxins are stored and become concentrated. This form of fat, when eaten incorrectly, can have no beneficial properties for the body other than adding fat to the waistline and around the arteries, but there is a way to enjoy it so continue reading to get the inside scoop.

- *Trans fat* - This is a type of fat that occurs naturally in some foods in small amounts. But most trans fats are made from oils through a food processing method called partial hydrogenation, which is basically all manufactured oils. By partially hydrogenating oils, they become easier to cook with and less likely to spoil than naturally occurring oils. Research studies show that these partially hydrogenated trans fats can increase unhealthy LDL cholesterol and lower healthy high-density lipoprotein (HDL) cholesterol. This can increase your risk of cardiovascular disease. Most fats that have a high percentage of saturated fat or that contain trans fats are solid at room temperature. Because of this, they're typically referred to as solid fats. They include beef fat, pork fat, butter, shortening and stick margarine.

There is only one challenge here, research from the *British Medical Journal*, *Annals of Internal Medicine*, the Weston Price Foundation and several others who have been involved in the studies of saturated fat have come to say that saturated fat has several beneficial factors for human health. We are more at risk from processed vegetable oils than a stick of butter. Once again, the main key here is all on the quality of our choices.

- Vitamins A, D, E, and K are actually found in saturated fat and can only be absorbed in the body with the use of fat.
- Saturated fats are a main initiator for the manufacturing of both testosterone and estrogen.
- Saturated fats are a critical component of the nervous system and assure the proper function of the nerves.
- Saturated fats help to reduce inflammation as long as they are consumed away from processed carbohydrates. When saturated fats are combined with flour and sugar, they produce an inflammatory response in the body. This is what made them so bad in the first place. The combination created an unhealthy response in the body. Consuming saturated fats away from flour and sugar actually reduces inflammation and provides the body with additional benefits. So watch out "cookie monsters"—yup, cookies are not your best choice. Personally, I make mine with cold-pressed coconut oil and a few other superfoods to

give my kids something healthy and tasty, but you will see more of this once we get to the recipe section.

🌳 The saturated fat components from both grass-fed butter and coconut oil actually strengthen the immune system and assist in cellular communication throughout the body. This in turn helps with cancer and several other health challenges.

There are still numerous benefits that are all attributed to fats in the diet. Cholesterol seems to be a big factor when it comes to fat, but it is important to understand that our bodies only manufacture cholesterol as a result of breaking down processed foods, not from gathering the cholesterol from foods that contain it. LDL, which is your "bad cholesterol", is manufactured as a byproduct of your body repairing itself from the damages of breaking down and metabolizing processed foods.

As with all foods, nutritional density is the key; choose fats that provide you with added nutrients and the body will reap the benefits. Processed fats and oils are lacking enzymes and have been altered from their natural state. Fats that are naturally derived from a food source with little to no processing can provide us with an array of benefits. Our top choices are: cold pressed coconut oil, cold pressed olive oil, organic grass-fed butter*, organic ghee, organic grass-fed meats, bone broth, unheated organic nut oils, avocados, raw nuts, and organic/pasture fed eggs—it's all about the QUALITY of your choices!

*I emphasize "Organic Grass Fed" because this actually changes the nutritional density of the butter or meat. When a cow is fed a processed meal, the nutrient content of that cow changes, pesticide residue increases, and the digestibility of the meat becomes more challenging. This leaves us with meat that increases our LDL, increases inflammation in the body, and provides little if any quality nutrition.

Good Fats (the following information is retrieved from The Mayo Clinic.org):

The types of potentially helpful dietary fat are mostly unsaturated:

> *Monounsaturated fat* - This is a type of fat is found in a variety of foods and oils. It is more liquid in nature, brings in several essential nutrients, and helps to protect our internal organs and acts as a lubricant for the body. Studies show that eating foods rich in monounsaturated fats (MUFAs) improves blood cholesterol levels, which can decrease your risk of heart disease. Research also shows that MUFAs may benefit insulin levels and blood sugar control, which can be especially helpful if you have type 2 diabetes. (**Keep in mind that fat will slow down the spike of sugar during digestion, this is why it aids in blood sugar control)

> *Polyunsaturated fat* - This is a type of fat found mostly in plant-based foods and oils. Evidence shows that eating foods rich in polyunsaturated fats (PUFAs) improves blood cholesterol levels, which can decrease your risk of heart disease. PUFAs may also help decrease the risk of type 2 diabetes.

> *Omega-3 fatty acid* - One type of polyunsaturated fat is made up of mainly omega-3 fatty acids and may be especially beneficial to your heart and brain. Omega-3,

found in some types of fatty fish, appears to decrease the risk of coronary artery disease. It may also protect against irregular heartbeats and help lower blood pressure levels. There are plant sources of omega-3 fatty acids; however, the body doesn't convert it and use it as well as omega-3 from fish. *Either way, think of these as the Power Foods of your child's brain development, the fuel that feeds the brain. These are an essential part of brain development and growth.*

Foods made up mostly of monounsaturated and polyunsaturated fats are liquid at room temperature, such as olive oil, coconut oil, and avocado oil (of course all of these are cold-pressed and unrefined). Fish high in omega-3 fatty acids include salmon, tuna, trout, mackerel, sardines and herring. Plant sources of omega-3 fatty acids include flaxseeds (ground and oil), raw nuts and other raw seeds (walnuts, nut butter, chia, hemp and sunflower).

Cholesterol: HDL is GOOD and LDL is BAD. The bottom line is that for most people cholesterol is produced in the body as a defense mechanism against arterial "scrapes". What is meant by this is that certain foods, such as corn syrup and high fructose corn syrup, are challenging to break down during the digestive process. They require so much effort that arteries are slightly damaged, initiating the body to produce cholesterol to repair the damage. With this said, foods only provoke your body to produce cholesterol; cholesterol from foods does not typically "stick" to your arteries during digestion. There are individuals with certain hereditary conditions that form excess cholesterol with and without the provoking foods, these individuals will have ongoing cholesterol issues and should be monitored closely by their physicians.

As you can see, everything seems to work together; it all depends on the quality of the food source as to the health benefits and energy distribution you receive. This next grouping of items is present in every carbohydrate, protein and even fat source you consume. Ideally, you want to receive all of the benefits of these directly from your foods. Nutrients work synergistically, so buying a specific nutrient at the store and receiving it directly from your food are really two different things. Foods will always give you a better, well-rounded level of nutrients that cannot be duplicated in a pill form (more on this in the Supplement Section).

Vitamins

These are the body's regulators that perform every internal action that is necessary to maintain life. They are a non-caloric, organic substance that can be classified as water soluble or fat soluble. Water soluble vitamins (such as B and C) are absorbed directly into the bloodstream. Fat soluble vitamins (such as A, D, E, and K) are stored in the fatty tissue of the body and require dietary fat for digestion and assimilation. The most common ones are:

A – Maintains the skin and mucous membrane and plays an integral part in the health of the eyes.

B – Maintains normal carbohydrate metabolism and assists with the energy centers of the body. (Side note for moms...helps us recuperate during times of stress.)

C – Primary antioxidant/immune booster, it is involved in most of the bodily functions and repair.

D – Assists the body in the absorption of calcium for bone health.

E – Assists the body in tissue repair.

K – Plays an integral part in blood clotting.

We need over 96 vitamins and minerals per day in order to have our bodies work at their very best. With fruits and vegetables, the darker the richer the color, the more nutrients they provide. Focus more on offering a rainbow of produce and your family will create a strong foundation of health.

Minerals

Essential Minerals are typically divided into two groups: Major Minerals (macro minerals) and Trace Minerals (micro minerals). Both of these are equally important and have specific responsibilities for the body's internal processes, yet trace minerals are commonly needed in smaller quantities than major minerals. They are both naturally occurring but inorganic in nature. A balanced diet usually provides all of the essential minerals. Some of the most common from each group are as follows:

Major Minerals

Sodium – Water distribution and nerve function

Phosphorus – Healthy bones & teeth, and energy prod.

Calcium – Teeth and bones

Potassium – Water in the blood and tissues

Trace Minerals

Iron – Helps red blood cells carry oxygen

Copper – Protects cells from damage

Zinc – Immunity and wound healing

Iodine – Thyroid gland function

Selenium – Protects cells

Chromium – Metabolism of carbohydrates, proteins, fats

The Secret Element of Food Success...

OK, so most of the boring stuff is now over, but there is one more thing that makes a huge difference in how we process and assimilate foods. Our body is designed to optimally function on quality fuel that provides vitamins, minerals and enzymes. Enzymes are like a computer code that tells our body specifically what to do with all of the components of that particular food; the key is that enzymes only survive in raw, unprocessed foods. For example: the enzymes of an apple will tell the body what to do with the vitamins, minerals, and fiber, and anything extra gets tossed from there. Enzymes are the magic compound of RAW Foods! They help the body in the following ways:

- They are needed for every chemical reaction of the body
- They're connected to every working organ of the body and run life's processes (including weight loss)
- They assist the body with detoxification and cleansing
- They break down foods and distribute nutrients to all needed locations of the body
- They help the body with the digestive process
- Enzymes are destroyed with heat (greater than 105 degrees) as in cooking and are non-existent in processed foods

Enzymes come in several varieties with numerous jobs throughout the body. Digestive enzymes are designed to help break down foods and assist the body's distribution system for nutrients, fiber, and the disposal of any unnecessary parts. In other words, food that is raw or has been heated at or below 105 degrees provides the body with an array of digestive enzymes that tell the body how to use and organize all of the compounds found in the foods eaten. Unfortunately, heat and processing kill off these valuable elements, making it harder for the body to organize all of the food compounds and making it easier to store those foods as fat.

Cooked foods rob our bodies of stored digestive enzymes, thus requiring more effort from our system to break down and digest our foods. This process progressively breaks down our system, creating digestive issues and malabsorption. Ideally, we would combine both raw and cooked foods in order to super charge our digestive process and utilize the enzymes from the raw foods to break down the cooked foods. This in turn would alleviate any digestive "distress" and assist our bodies in fully digesting and utilizing all of the wonderful properties of those foods.

Without enzymes:

1. Foods can be easily stored as fat.

2. Nutrients are robed from body reserves for digestion.

It's all pretty simple, the more we focus on quality foods in their natural, unprocessed, state, the less we need to focus on calories. Your job is to encourage your family to eat for the nutritional value of their foods, to gain strength from the nutrients and build muscle from the protein.

Water

This is the major element for all of the workings of the human body. Water is a critical element of the body, and adequate hydration is a must to allow the body to function. Up to 75% of the body's weight is made up of water. Most of the water is found within the cells of the body, known as intracellular space; this is the primary carrier of nutrients. The rest is found in the extracellular space, which consists of the blood vessels (intravascular space) and the spaces between cells (interstitial space). Water is responsible for the removal of metabolic byproducts and toxins that are in the body. Water works side by side with the liver to metabolize fat efficiently through cardiovascular training and works directly in the muscle to assist muscular contraction for strength gain. A decrease in water leads to dehydration and for any active child that can mean anything from fatigue to muscle breakdown and even a reduction in fat-burning capability. As the demand for water increases, through exercise, heat, and general exertion, the consumption must also increase.

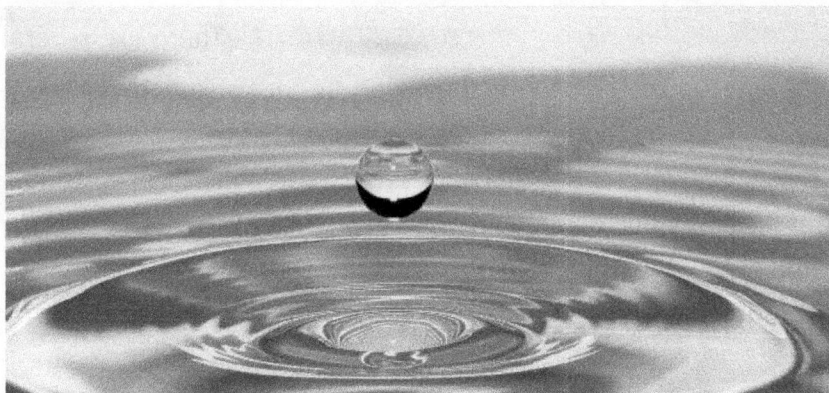

As with nutritional needs, water is very specific to body weight, activity level, and the lean muscle mass of the individual. The average individual should follow these guidelines:

- Minimum of 8 glasses of H_2O a day for an adult and 6 for a child
- Add 2 more glasses of H_2O for any beverage that contains alcohol or caffeine (hopefully the kids aren't indulging in these, just saying).
- Rate your hydration by the color of your urine (clear is optimal)

When the body lacks water, it sends out the feeling of thirst; if that is not addressed then the next alarm becomes hunger. Hunger can be a facade for thirst, the body will send out this signal in hopes of extracting fluids from the food. Caffeine, alcohol and certain medications can also contribute to dehydration. Of course, these should never be used for children, but for you adults you need to understand how these substances can increase dehydration. They should be kept to a minimum; but if consumed, extra amounts of water will help to counterbalance the effects.

Alternative Water Substitutes - There are several different waters out there that promise vitamins and minerals, electrolyte replacements, and the like. These are all synthetically derived and without the proper synergistic balance of nutrients and enzymes our bodies will not receive all of the benefits they sell us on. With this said the best substitute for water is raw coconut water.

Coconut water is an isotonic solution, which replaces the fluids and minerals that the body loses during physical activities. For this reason, many athletes and individuals who work out regularly are encouraged to drink coconut water to replace all the minerals and fluids they lose while working out. Even the United Nations Food and Agriculture Organization (FAO) attested to the benefits of drinking coconut water when it fought for a patent in 2000 to market it as the next big sports drinks.

Basically, coconut water is like natural Gatorade. It contains water, simple carbohydrates (or sugars), naturally occurring enzymes, and electrolytes (or minerals). Sports drinks are made with refined sugars, artificial flavoring, synthetically derived nutrients, and food coloring, all of which can wreak havoc on a child's temperament, energy, and mood. With that said, I'd say coconut water represents a solid upgrade.

How Does This Come Together?

The components above form the essence of all human function and are absorbed into our bodies through the digestive process. That process begins the moment we put food or liquids into our mouth. Digestive enzymes begin to break down the food into its own unique components and water distributes them throughout the body to the areas that need them the most. This absorption of nutrients gives us the energy to exercise and the strength to maintain a healthy body free from illness and disease. Everything we consume has a nutritional value, some more than others; this helps to enhance the health of our bodies. As a society we have been programmed to eat for comfort, socialization or simply for fun. Our bodies are very intelligent and if they get the appropriate level of nutrients they function at a top level. Many of us make food choices that lack the nutrients we need, so our bodies scream out, "I'm Hungry!" and we keep eating until that one vitamin we are craving is located. Your body is like a fine-tuned automobile and if you fill it with high quality premium fuel and take good care of it, it will perform like never before. On the other hand, if you fill it with low grade fuel and skip the tune up here and there, it will move in a low grade manner, sluggish and unmotivated to perform!

As your family's food coach you want to instill the benefits of high quality foods, encouraging everyone to look for nutritionally dense foods that reward the body with good health. Remember that 200 calories of pizza is not equal to 200 calories of sautéed vegetables and fish. You may be providing your body with its caloric energy needs, but the lack of nutrients will make the body desire more food until its nutritional needs have been met. Once your body is fulfilled with high quality foods, its need and desires for lower quality foods will dissipate. It is all about developing the pallet of your family and creating a pallet that craves higher quality foods and can easily pass on lower quality "knock offs".

As individuals we all metabolize foods differently and due to our individual biochemistry we all have very individual nutritional needs. The one thing that is clear is that the food choices we make can add to our health or add to weight gain, weight loss, moodiness, inability to concentrate, and a host of additional health related issues. You want to give your family the knowledge to make wiser choices that will enhance their health and wellbeing. You want to teach them how to make quality choices without feeling deprived, left out or on a "diet" of sorts. This is about a Lifetime Food Plan, about eating for whole food nutrition, and about creating the right food plan that can be easily executed and enjoyed.

So, no matter what age we are dealing with, we all need good quality fats and proteins combined with carbohydrates from fruits and vegetables to stabilize our energy. The more time that lapses in between meals the higher the amount of protein and fats we should include. This formula will keep you satiated, focused, clear-headed and energized. When processed foods and simple carbohydrates from sugar, flour, and dairy are thrown in the mix, they slow us down, fog the mind, and distract our thoughts. These should only be an occasional treat, more than that and they will throw us out of whack and create more harm than good. This is a pretty straightforward formula that works for all ages.

As parents we strive for our children to learn, enjoy, and create a strong immune system for life. Simple carbohydrates from sugar, flour, and dairy as well as processed foods will take you further and further away from your objectives and they ALL break down as a sugar. So here you are giving a child "mac and

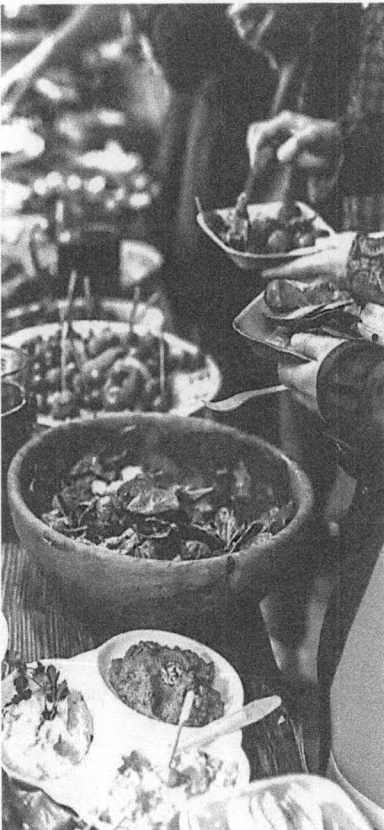

cheese"; it's a common food among children, but guess what, it breaks down as a sugar, there is very little protein and fat to stabilize their blood sugar. Too many sugars in the diet encourage weight gain, inattentiveness, and lethargy, not to mention additional sugar cravings. I realize this can seem very overwhelming and, depending on how your current household food plan is laid out, you may have some work to do. No matter where you are today, change can happen; it is all about taking it one step at a time.

"I remember taking my son to a playgroup, at a school, to see if it would be something he would like. He was two at the time. Snacks arrived right when we got there and the teachers offered the kids a bag of fruit loops and half a bagel. My son wasn't having any of that and shortly after, we had a room filled with wild bangies and my son crawled up on my lap wanting to go home."

Notes, Stuff to Remember, Things to Buy, etc.

Myths and Misconceptions

On my quest to clear up the food confusions that are out there, I would like to clarify a few misconceptions to help you have a better understanding when choosing the right foods for your family. The food industry has become a multi-million dollar industry with branches of it even receiving additional revenue from pesticide and pharmaceutical companies. There are several tactics used to excite us to purchase various items that do more harm than good. The key to all of this is to learn as much as possible so that you can be your own health advocate and so that you can make the best possible choices without depending on a store, company or manufacturer to be looking after your best interest.

Interpreting a Food Label

Here are a few ways that the Food Label can hide some important information:

1. Calories per serving – What you consider a serving and what the food industry considers a serving are two different things. Be sure to understand what the

serving size looks like compared to your serving size.

2. All of the % values are based on a 2000-calorie diet; your children are not eating 2000 calories, so these values are not very helpful for you.

3. Remember that what the food label says and how your body metabolizes it are two totally different things. Something with zero fat grams can still be stored as fat. Additionally, since flour and dairy will break down as a sugar, consider your total carbohydrates equal to the amount of sugar that your body will take in, not just the sugar total alone.

4. The DV% represents the % of the recommended allowance total for a specific nutrient, but it is still figured out using a 2000 calorie diet.

"The other day my client presented me with her favorite, organic, super yummy cereal. She claimed it was low calorie and just wanted my seal of approval. Upon reading the food label it was 120 calories per serving. A serving size is ¼ cup, this part she did not realize. When we measured her serving size it was a cup and a half...600 calories for breakfast, OMG!"

Serving Size ①

Nutrition Facts

Serving Size 1 cup (253 g)
Servings Per Container 4

Amount Per Serving	
Calories 260	Calories from Fat 72

Calories ②

	% Daily Value*
Total Fat 8g	13%
Saturated Fat 3g	17%
Cholesterol 130mg	44%
Sodium 1010mg	42%
Total Carbohydrate 22g	7%
Dietary Fiber 9g	36%
Sugars 4g	
Protein 25g	

List of Nutrients ③

% Daily Value ④

Vitamin A	35%	•	Vitamin C	2%
Calcium	6%	•	Iron	30%

Vitamins & Minerals ⑤

* Percent Daily Values are based on a 2,000 calorie diet. Your daily values may be higher or lower depending on your calorie needs.

	Calories	2,000	2,500
Total Fat	Less than	65g	80g
Sat Fat	Less than	20g	25g
Cholesterol	Less than	300mg	300mg
Sodium	Less than	2,400mg	2,400mg
Total Carbohydrate		300g	375g
Fiber		25g	30g

Daily Values ⑥

Calories per gram:
Fat 9 • Carbohydrate 4 • Protein 4

Calories Per Gram ⑦

INGREDIENTS:

Filtered Water, Organic Maltodextrin, Organic Evaporated Cane Sugar, Natural Flavors, Dipotassium Phosphate, Salt, Magnesium Citrate, Calcium Lactate, Monkfruit.

Now look at the following ingredient lists. Ingredients are listed in descending order of weight (from most to least). Note that anything below 10% of the total ingredients does not need to be listed on the ingredient list. Manufacturers can hide many unhealthy items under the premise of "Natural Flavors"; this could mean anything from MSG to an array of preservatives. Also, as long at 30% of the ingredients are organic, they can sell the product as "organic". With this said, all ingredients would need to say "organic" and those that don't ... are not.

There are various names used to list sugar, MSG, preservatives or chemical derivatives. So here is how I handle it... If you cannot pronounce something on the ingredient list and don't know what it is—Don't Eat It!

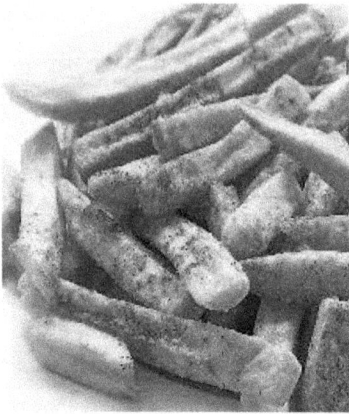

Potatoes, canola oil, hydrogenated soybean oil, safflower oil, natural flavor (vegetable Source), dextrose, sodium acid, pyrophosphate (maintain color), citric acid (preservative), dimethylopolysiloxane (antifoaming agent), and cooked in vegetable oil (canola oil, corn oil, soybean oil, hydrogenated soybean oil with THBQ, citric acid, dimethylpolysiloxane), and salt (sillicoaluminate, dextrose, potassium iodide)

Manufactured and processed foods bring with them more challenges than benefits. Manufacturers have mastered the art of deception in both their packaging and ingredient terminology, making it even more important to understand ingredients and how they affect health.

Packaging Claims

Packaged and processed foods are filled with a variety of claims and marketing "words" to make you excited about your purchase. Many of these nutritional claims are false. For example, "light" vegetable oil is merely light in color, and "light" cheesecake light in texture. With new labeling, any term used to describe a particular food's nutrient content will have a universal meaning. Unfortunately, the food label can contain just a few ingredients that fit the claim and still highlight it on the packaging. Such words as "organic", "non-GMO", "natural", "free", "low," "light or lite," "less," and "high" may or may not be listed correctly.

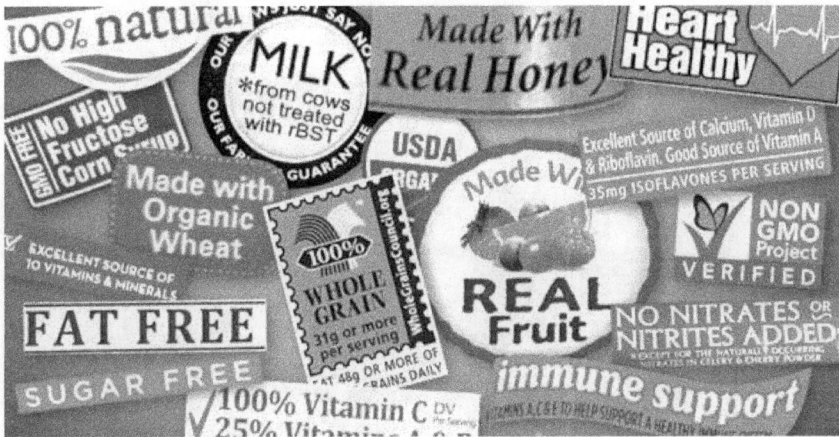

Only under certain circumstances can claims link a nutrient or a food to the risks of disease. The January 6, 1993 issue of the *Federal Register* permits the following nutrient-health relationships:

- Calcium and reduced risk of osteoporosis
- Dietary fiber and reduced risk of certain cancers

- Sodium and increased risk of hypertension
- Dietary saturated fat and cholesterol and increased risk of coronary heart disease
- Dietary fat and increased risk of certain cancers

These regulations allow information on food labels that can help educate the public about recognized diet-disease relationships. Authorized claims must meet requirements to prevent label information that would be false or misleading. The FDA and USDA have begun a multi-year labeling education campaign designed to increase consumer knowledge and to help consumers make accurate and sound dietary choices. Check out www.Greenerchoices.org for a comprehensive explanation of over 150 governmental and third-party food labels.

Produce Codes Unveiled

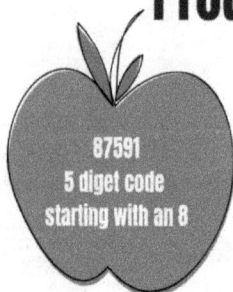

87591
5 diget code
starting with an 8

4011
4 diget code
starting with a 3 or 4

934021
5 diget code
starting with a 9

GENETICALLY MODIFIED

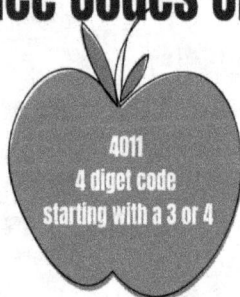

CONVENTIONAL

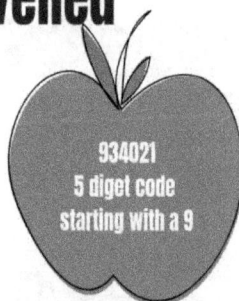

ORGANIC

Organics

This has been the catchphrase for some time now, it basically means that no pesticides were used to grow these foods and that no chemicals were added to the food during processing. With so many health issues coming to light, it's best to provide our bodies with as few chemicals as possible. The research is limited, but there is evidence that organics are farmed in such a manner that the soils are not depleted and the nutritional levels are higher than their conventional counterparts. On the flip side, many argue that organic farms still receive residue from both GMO and pesticides, most farms take the utmost care to assure the quality of their grains or produce. Either way, the levels of any possible chemical will be much less on an organic farm than a conventional one.

Organic vs. Conventional – Conventional fruits and vegetables are sprayed down with varying levels of pesticides that have been deemed safe by the FDA on studies performed on an average 150 lb. adult male. The pesticides penetrate the produce through the outer layer, so those with thicker skins (i.e. oranges, bananas) may contain lower levels than those with thin or no skins (i.e. strawberries, raspberries). Organic produce is produce that has been grown in soils that have been re-cultivated to have no pesticide residue and are grown without the use of any pesticides. These are usually much pricier than conventional produce but tend to have a higher nutritional value.

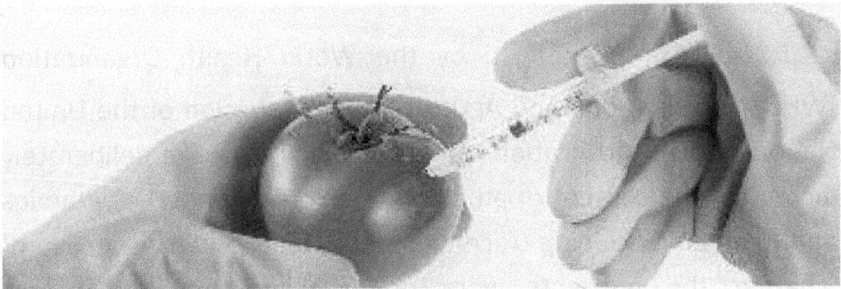

Genetically Modified Foods

(GMO or engineered foods) — Although this is a fairly new phenomenon, the pesticide industry has genetically modified seeds from such crops as sugar beets, corn, soy, and wheat. They have engineered these seeds to withstand high levels of pesticides without killing the crop or modified the seed to carry its own internal pesticide so that when the bug tries to eat the plant, the bug dies. The FDA does not require vendors to list ingredients that have been engineered, although some vendors are proud to list that there is "No GMO" in their products. Are these safe choices or not? Research is limited and with mixed reviews; unfortunately, the research that does promote GMO typically originates from the pesticide companies or the conventional farmers that use them.

"When ingredients are organic and wholesome, your body has the best chance of absorbing the good nutrition it provides. When a scientist adds it in, your body has to decide if it wants to use it or not, and most of the time it will choose healthy food options as opposed to "healthy manufactured options".

Fortified - As defined by the World Health Organization (WHO) and the Food and Agricultural Organization of the United Nations (FAO), fortification refers to "the practice of deliberately increasing the content of an essential micronutrient, i.e. vitamins and minerals (including trace elements), in a food irrespective of whether the nutrients were originally in the food before processing or not, so as to improve the nutritional quality of the food supply and to provide a public health benefit with minimal risk to health," whereas enrichment is defined as "synonymous with fortification" and refers to the addition of micronutrients to a food that were lost during processing. 80+ years ago, fortification of foods was started to enrich the nutrient content of foods in countries where malnutrition was prevalent.

To break this down even further, this initially started with foods sent over to impoverished nations as a means of enhancing their nutrients in a "processed food" delivery system. Since they were vitamin deficient from the start, their bodies reveled in the flood of nutrients they were receiving. Today, no matter how badly we eat, we still receive enough nutrients for survival. With this said, "fortified" foods actually provide us with no great benefit except for calories, since our bodies have a hard time assimilating synthetically derived nutrients and would rather wait and receive them from a natural source. The challenge with us is that we are not malnourished so the synthetic nutrients are rarely absorbed by our systems.

http://www.who.int/nutrition/publications/guide_food_fortificati on_micronutrients.pdf

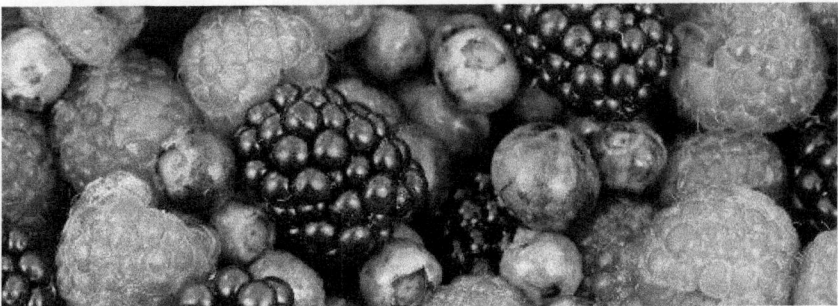

Superfoods

This relatively new term refers to foods that have large amounts of nutrition per bite or have a high nutritional density. www.eatrightamerica.com rates the superfoods by an ERNI Score; some markets use an ANDI Score—either way this helps us identify which fruits or vegetables to choose from for a higher nutritional punch. Here are my Top Ten Favorites to choose from:

Kale

Collard Greens

Hemp Seeds

Chia Seeds

Quinoa

Coconut Products

Berries

Avocado

Raw Walnuts

Pomegranate

Essential Fatty Acids (EFAs)

Feed the brain RIGHT! For our kids this means that their growing brains will receive all the nourishment needed, and for adults it will keep our brains intact for years to come. So what are the best sources?

Eggs - but not just from any chicken, you want Organic, Free Range, and Pasture Fed.

Raw Hemp Seeds - This complete protein has little taste and can be easily combined into a salad, smoothie or anything else you can dream of and your kids won't even know it's there.

Raw Flax Seeds - These can also be added to just about anything but should be freshly ground before eating and stored in the fridge or freezer.

Salmon or Sardines - These are the "crown jewels", our bodies assimilate these best. Our challenge is finding sources that are not farmed and are caught swimming wild and free.

Raw Nuts, *especially Walnuts* - Raw nut butters or freshly-chopped nuts can be added to just about anything, and don't forget a handful of trail mix, that's a good option as well! Keep in mind that your traditional peanut butter does not go in this category. Since it is roasted it loses most of the valuable nutrients that are available when it is raw. Unfortunately, peanut butter is kind of "icky" raw so your best bet is one of the amazing alternative raw nut butters out there.

Avocados - This poor fruit has had a bad rap of being fatty - No limits, just enjoy and reap all of the nutritional benefits it provides you with. This may sound odd, but avocado smashed up with a banana makes for an excellent baby food treat!

Supplements

They are just that, they supplement the body in order to provide missing nutrients that the body is not receiving from foods. Ideally you should receive everything from your foods, which is one of the main reasons why it is so important to include a large variety of fruits and vegetables. As your family's food coach you want to make sure that everyone is receiving all of the colors of the rainbow from their fruits and vegetables; if for some reason a nutritional deficiency is suspected then that's when you bring in a qualified professional who will take a blood, stool or urine sample to find out specifically what is missing and formulate a plan to best resolve any deficiencies.

Many nutritional supplements have been promoted to increase performance, maximize fat burning or even enhance energy. Unfortunately, without the right information, the ingredients can have adverse reactions with medications. There is no quick resolve for fat loss and no health benefits from stimulants. Many athletes of all ages feel compelled to try the latest and greatest in hopes of reaping the rewards that they may or may not provide. Here is a brief list of some of the top choices out there to give you an idea of what they do. Just remember that if any of your family members want to try a supplement for some type of physical benefit, it's a good idea to bring in a professional to be sure to choose the right one for the right needs.

Ergogenic Aids and Energy Enhancement Supplements – These are a supplement that addresses performance and energy. Most of these provide unhealthy levels of caffeine and/or other stimulants.

Protein Powder – In a quest to increase their dietary protein, many are looking to a quick resolve through a powder or protein type drink. These, as with all supplements, should be left to a qualified professional who is better adept at prescribing the best product to meet the needs of the client. The average individual's protein needs can easily be achieved with foods. Not all protein powders are bad, if you want to sneak some into a smoothie, pancake or even a muffin there are several raw plant based protein powders that are minimally processed and can be a great addition to a family food plan (see the recipe section for more information).

Protein Bars – This industry has taken over the candy bar market. In general they provide protein, some synthetically derived vitamins and minerals, but most are heavily packed with sugar and may or may not include some form of energy stimulant. There are several quality bars out there that are minimally processed; it's a matter of reading the food label to decide which bar works best. Many of the Raw Food Bar types can be a great "emergency food" plan when on the road with the kids. They will provide a decent amount of protein and quality nutrients as opposed to any fast food choices you would find out and about.

Sweeteners

This refers to everything from sugar to stevia, agave, and more, but it is important to recognize that many other things metabolize as a sugar and when too much "sugar" is being processed it is then stored as FAT and can enhance mental distractions and energy levels for kids. The average consumer consumes 22 teaspoons of sugar per day; the body can safely handle 6 teaspoons of sugar per day. For discussion purposes this section will only discuss sweeteners, but keep in mind that sugar, flour, and dairy (and for you adults, this would include alcohol as well) all break down as a sugar so when you combine sweeteners with flour and dairy, you add even more sugar into the system.

Hidden terms referring to sugar: There are over 100 names for sugar that are used by manufacturers to hide the fact that they are adding a ton of sugar to your foods. They use such names as malt barley, molasses, brown rice syrup, cane juice, carob syrup, dextran, diastatic malt, and many more to make you believe these are natural ingredients or preservatives.

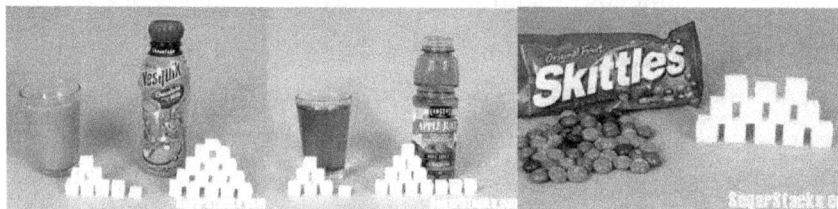

SugarStacks.com does a great job in illustrating the amount of sugar in many popular foods. I love to use these illustrations with kids so they can clearly see what it is all about. Keep in mind that these illustrations only represent sugar, not the flour and dairy component.

The following are the most common types of sugar and their effects on our health:

Table Sugar (sucrose) – Typically manufactured from sugar beets (which is on the top 5 list of GMO foods). Table sugar is a combination of fructose and glucose (glucose being what we use for energy), and although it provides less fructose than HFCS it can break down easier but still with a variety of health concerns. There is no nutritional benefit to table sugar.

Corn Syrup and High Fructose Corn Syrup (HFCS) – These sweeteners are addictive, inexpensive to make, and metabolize as a fructose, which causes stress to the liver. Fructose is turned into free fatty acids (FFAs), VLDL (the damaging form of cholesterol), and triglycerides, which get stored as fat and trigger high cholesterol. Additionally, these sweeteners have been linked to high cholesterol, heart disease, diabetes, and obesity. And guess what? A lot of food manufacturers love using these types with packaged kids' foods because they can easily get the kids "hooked" on it, so expect to see this in everything from candy to pasta sauce and so much more.

Agave – This is a highly processed sap from a cactus that is *almost all fructose*. Your blood sugar will spike just as it would if you were consuming regular sugar or HFCS. Agave's rise in popularity is due to a great marketing campaign, but any health benefits present in the original agave plant are processed out.

**Stevia* – This is a tea leaf. And when steeped as a tea, it produces a naturally sweet liquid that can be used as a sweetener for just about anything. The challenge arises when it has been over processed and no longer looks like a "tea". With this said, liquid stevia is your best choice; it should have no chemical additives, it naturally has no calories and few, if any, side effects.

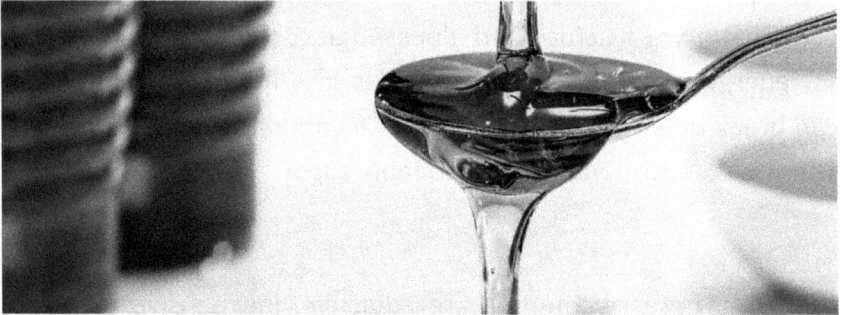

**Honey* - This blend of sugar, trace enzymes, minerals, vitamins, and amino acids is quite unlike any other sweetener and brings along an entire list of healthful benefits. Honey still breaks down as a fructose, but its combination of enzymes, healing and antibacterial properties makes it a much better choice.

**These are the two best choices when it comes to health, calories, and any nutritional benefits.

Other things to know about SUGAR:

Did you know your immune system can be placed on SNOOZE? With only 8 teaspoons of traditional table sugar, corn syrup, high fructose corn syrup or the like, your immune system can be suppressed up to 40% for 30 minutes all the way to 5 hours. So … better think twice before indulging with that soda or candy bar or anything else that satisfies your sweet tooth. Remember: Sugar, flour, and dairy ALL metabolize as a sugar. So next time a teacher gives your child a piece of candy, put your foot down. School is the last place someone needs candy from, between losing focus and suppressing the immune system, it's not worth it at all!

How fast does the sugar get into your system? The Glycemic Index is a measure of how quickly a food will increase blood sugar. Simple sugars, such as high fructose corn syrup, quickly flood the blood with fructose and glucose. This puts stress on the body, which attempts to bring blood sugar back to equilibrium. The lower the Glycemic Index the slower the blood sugar will rise. These foods have more protein, fiber, and/or fat in order to slow down the digestive process. With a high Glycemic Index, foods that are not immediately used for energy are easily stored as fat. A good example of this is a banana; if you eat the banana and work out, the sugar will be used for the workout and the nutrients absorbed in the body. Now if you eat a banana, a cookie, and a bowl of pasta and just sit back for the day, there is too much sugar in the system and the body will store much of the unused content as fat.

Salt

Salt is not a terrible thing. The challenge has been the numerous choices that we are surrounded with. Traditional table salt provides the body with no nutritional value and actually strips us of needed nutrients just so the body can metabolize it. Choose salts like Celtic sea salt or Himalayan salt; these taste the same as table salt but are packed with naturally occurring enzymes, minerals and vitamins to keep the body in optimal condition.

Chicken and Meat

Do you buy Hormone Free, Natural, or Organic or do you choose the best deal in the store?

FYI – if you choose to do neither, your meat or chicken is probably packed with growth hormone and/or antibiotics and they are fed grains that include fillers and genetically modified ingredients. If this hasn't convinced you to go "Organic" yet, would this sound appealing? Arsenic, antibiotics, growth hormones, pesticides, and whatever else is available to enhance the quality and appearance of ... conventional chicken. We realize cost may be a factor, but if you educate yourself enough and understand the quality of various food items, you'll be able to choose organic for the things that could affect the health of you and your family and choose conventional for the rest.

Organic – This means that no drugs were used on the animals and that all the feed is clean of pesticides or genetically modified crops. The key here is to also recognize if they are vegetarian fed or naturally fed.

Free Range, Organic, Grass or Pasture Fed – This is the "mecca" of fine poultry and meat. These are organic, they roam freely in their natural environment, and they eat from their natural food source without any alterations.

Natural – The animals were fed natural grains with no fillers or byproducts, but the grains are not organic and they are more than likely genetically modified. Also, unless otherwise specified, these could have been given hormones and/or antibiotics.

Hormone /Antibiotic Free – This simply means that they used no drugs to "plump" up the meat or produce extra milk. With chickens they used no drugs to "plump" up the chicken or to produce more eggs than natural. Also no antibiotics were used to kill off bacteria, etc.

Wild Game – Sounds intimidating, but it is one of the better bets. These are free roaming animals, no drugs, they eat their natural diet, and they run free. They are mainly sold from specialty ranches across the country and are packaged without any additional preservatives or chemicals that you would find in the grocery store. Check out this site for some wonderful meats and more information http://www.brokenarrowranch.com/. (Try Boneless Loin- Axis Venison, it is mighty tasty!)

Fish

Fish provides a wonderful amount of protein and an ideal amount of Essential Fatty Acids; unfortunately, mercury and PCBs puts a damper on many of our choices. Mercury's toxicity can take up to a year to leave the system. According to the U.S. Environmental Protection Agency, a safe level of mercury consumption is 1.51 micrograms per day. The average can of tuna contains 52.7 micrograms of mercury per gram. The best situation is to include small amounts of fish in your family's food plan as opposed to utilizing fish as your main source of protein. Some of the health effects include impaired neurological development in the fetus, cancer, impairment of the peripheral vision, disturbances in sensations, lack of coordination of movements, Alzheimer's, impairment of speech, hearing, walking, and muscle weakness. Shrimp, canned light tuna, salmon, pollock, and catfish contain small amounts of mercury, but larger fish such as shark, swordfish, king mackerel, tuna steak or tilefish contain the highest levels of mercury and should be avoided. One more thing to keep in mind with fish is that "farm raised" means they are basically living and breeding in their own "stuff". Ideally there is wild farmed, these have moving water but are still fed a manufactured meal. On the other hand, WILD is really the best option and, although we are dealing with polluted waters and other toxins, there are some great benefits to be had from fish as long as it is only a small part of your food plan.

Dairy (milk, cheese, yogurt, etc.)

As mentioned in the sugar section of this book, dairy metabolizes or "breaks down" as a sugar. The majority of dairy products in the USA are pasteurized, which means they have been heated at very high temperatures to kill off any so-called "bacteria".

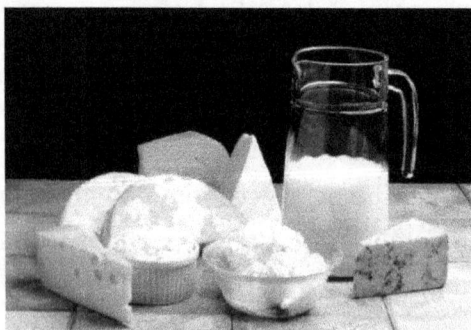

Unfortunately, this also kills off some of the amazing nutrients and enzymes that dairy provides. Most dairy is "fortified" with nutrients by a chemist and provides little if any protein. If chosen as a food source it should be eaten in small portions more as a treat than a main staple. And as for calcium, you get more calcium from a handful of almonds than you do a glass of milk, not to mention the other wonderful foods out there that give you quality calcium as well! Most children do better with an array of foods for their calcium needs than depending solely on dairy.

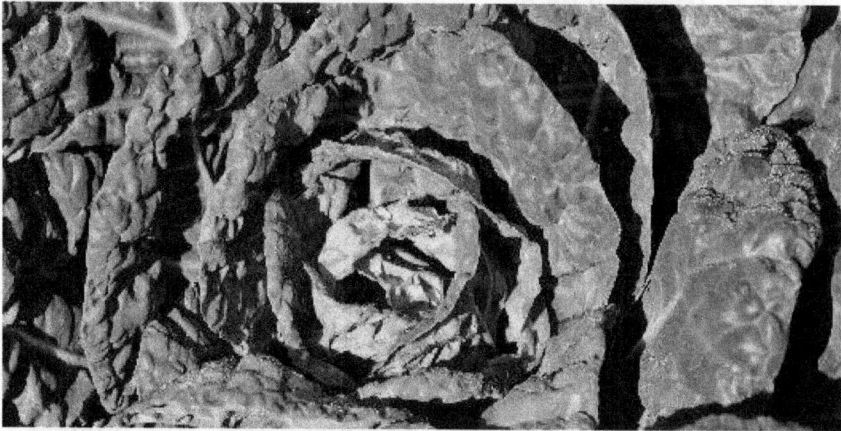

Leafy Greens

How many greens have you had today? Yes, greens—green, leafy vegetables that are packed with essential nutrients, fiber, and protein. If you can't get in that salad, try mixing in some kale or collard greens next time you make a smoothie. It may sound strange, but it's a great way to pack in the nutrients, and with the right amount of fruit you won't even know it's there! Just tell your kids it's an Incredible Hulk drink; get creative, make it sweet and they will never know the difference! But definitely don't limit yourself there; ground beef, marinara sauce, and so many other dishes are a great place to "hide" these treasured foods.

Intestinal Health

This has become a huge business these days; processed foods have disrupted our intestinal flora and made way for a breeding ground of bad bacteria and more. Pediatricians love to prescribe antibiotics, and unfortunately with repeated use this adds to our gut problems.

Probiotics, on the other hand, is the "good bacteria" and it assists the body in combating the bad bacteria and bringing back health to the digestive track. A healthy digestive tract will assist the body in assimilating all of the wonderful nutrients from our foods and disposing of all the "yucky" things we don't need. The average person should go to the bathroom 1–3 times per day; if that isn't happening, we need to talk. You can supplement your probiotics or you can add fermented foods and beverages such as kimchee, sauerkrauts or kombucha.

Caffeine

This comes in a variety of forms from sodas to coffee and anything in between. There has been some documentation as to its benefits during cardiovascular activity to improve the fat-burning system for adults, but it causes a great deal of dehydration and should be counterbalanced with additional glasses of water. Caffeine can be taxing on the system and can easily distract the mind. It causes challenges with the adrenal glands and the body's energy systems. Caffeine creates a false sense of energy and if overused can cause the body to reach a level of exhaustion that is hard to fix. For adults we need to get ourselves to a point where we don't NEED caffeine, we use it for those times where we have overdone ourselves and need a bit of a pick-me-up but not where we can't live without it. For children there is no need for caffeine, unfortunately it just starts messing with their adrenal glands before their time and creates additional unnecessary energy that can affect concentration and learning retention.

Adrenal Glands

Did you know that your adrenal glands are your "energy regulators"? These glands can provide you with unlimited energy throughout the day as long as you take good care of them. The best way to do this is to get adequate rest at night and avoid foods and beverages that provide a "false sense of energy", such as flour, sugar, dairy, alcohol, and caffeine. That's right, that bagel may be altering your energy level for your entire day. Since flour, dairy, and sugar all metabolize like a sugar they create a type of "energy spike" and, depending on how much sugar is involved, will determine how high that spike gets. With each spike comes a fall, and some falls are bigger than others. You should have an even amount of energy throughout the day. If you find yourself falling asleep at your desk around that 3:00 p.m. hour or your kids are having challenges focusing in class, the adrenal glands may be sleeping on the job and looking for a bit of TLC. For more information on Adrenal Fatigue http://www.adrenalfatigue.org/about-adrenal-fatigue.html

Notes, Stuff to Remember, Things to Buy, etc.

Dieting and Fat Loss

Dieting

The media continues to inundate the public with confusing and contradicting information about diets and dieting. For years a high protein, low carbohydrate diet was considered the best way to lose weight. Recent evidence suggests that everyone is different and that we all have our own unique metabolism and combination of foods that works for us. Evidence also suggests that it is healthier to maintain a small weight loss, rather than repeatedly taking off and putting on weight (yo-yo dieting). The speculation is that every time a person loses and gains weight, more body fat remains and more lean muscle mass is lost. For adults we live with weight challenges that possibly stemmed from childhood, during puberty you are set with a specific number of fat cells that you will live with for the rest of your life. Yup, so that skinny kid has the best chances of keeping their weight at bay during adulthood.

As parents we need to take responsibility of our families' food. Kids will eat all sorts of things out and about, but the home should be a sanctuary, a place that nurtures the healthy pallet and encourages nutritionally dense choices. Ideally we never want to place ourselves in the position of having to put a child on a diet, if fed the right foods a child's body will develop accordingly. Too many manufactured or processed foods will add unnecessary weight to a child and affect their self-esteem, peer interactions, and ultimately their grades.

Not All Calories Are Created Equal

According to the Merriam-Webster Dictionary, "a calorie is a unit of heat used to indicate the amount of energy that foods will produce in the human body." The only caveat here is that not all calories create the same response in the body. Many times our body will keep "asking" for calories, not because it is hungry but because it is nutritionally starved.

Traditionally a decrease in calories and increase in physical activity would be the weight loss plan of choice. One pound of weight is about 3,500 calories. Unfortunately, these measures did not take into consideration the quality of one's foods. If you concentrate on increasing nutritionally dense foods, paying little to no attention to the calorie count, you have a better chance of losing permanent weight or never putting the weight on in the first place. The old standards of reducing daily intake by 250 calories would result in a loss of approximately one half pound per week, but it would be substantially easier to gain that ½ lb.+ back. Severe caloric restriction and overtraining can reduce metabolism, making weight loss more difficult. Although caloric restriction is often chosen above exercise as a means of weight loss, incorporating a nutritionally dense food plan with exercise is the most effective for permanent weight loss. Exercise and food both rev up the metabolism and, when combined appropriately, can create a fat-burning machine.

Lifelong Diet Plan

It is important to understand that any diet that is not a lifelong plan will typically result in weight challenges. As your family's food coach you have the POWER to teach every member of your family how to enjoy a lifelong plan of health and wellness. You can encourage the habits that keep them lean and be the role model that they want to follow. A person who goes on a diet and loses weight but never addresses the issues that made them gain weight in the first place will eventually gain the weight back. We have been programed by our parents and society that food is pleasure, comfort, and something we deserve. Food is nourishment and health, it is "fuel", and that is all!

Many of us live our lives with a deep-seated psychological "crutch" that neither dieting nor exercise can resolve. This is where counseling can help us understand our relationship with food and readjust our thoughts to bring them back to a healthy food plan and lifestyle. On another note, our bodies are extremely intelligent and they do not take well to the feeling of starvation, either from calories or nutrients. Your body will work hard to keep you at your current weight, with the belief that anything below this would lead to "starvation". This is why a person who goes on a very strict or drastic weight loss program will gain the weight back plus a few extra pounds, and with time these extra pounds are even harder to remove. Your body puts these on as a buffer so that it will have a "reserve" of fat and nutrients just in case you "starve" it again. For adults this can be a very challenging situation to reverse, for a child it is even worse.

Most individuals feel that they need a very structured weight loss program. These commercial programs are usually calorically driven and the quality of foods is rarely emphasized. This is a challenge because the weight loss will only be a temporary thing and true lifelong food planning will not be addressed. Here is where you can step in to educate and promote whole food eating.

Common Dieting Philosophies and Challenges

As the advocate for your family's health and wellbeing it is a good idea to understand some of the common food philosophies so that you can have a better understanding. In today's society many families follow various eating styles; by understanding a few of the top ones you can clearly help your family decipher what they may experience at others' homes or what they hear about from many of their peers at school.

Vegetarian – Although there are several different kinds of vegetarians, the common philosophy here is that they do not eat meat and survive primarily on fruits, vegetables, grains, and nuts. Your biggest challenge as your family's food coach is the amount of protein that they consume in a day. If their energy levels are low or inconsistent, their intake of high quality protein may be minimal and this will need to be addressed. Your primary protein sources would come from raw nuts and seeds, quinoa, leafy greens, and beans. Some vegetarians will eat fish and eggs, which helps out even more. Is it bad for a child to choose this route? Not at all, but one thing is for sure, their pallet and food choices will continually change, so try to work with them, giving them a place to develop with the right set of guidelines.

Raw Foodist – One of the newer categories to a food plan, these individuals are vegetarian with the exception that they do not cook any of their foods and consume them all in a "raw" state. So with this they have the same challenges as a vegetarian—if their energy levels are low or inconsistent, their intake of high quality protein may be minimal and this will need to be addressed.

Macrobiotics – These individuals believe in eating primarily grains and supplementing with fruits, vegetables, nuts, and animal proteins. They also rarely consume processed foods. With this group it all depends on their sources of protein. If they are taking in a sufficient amount, their diet should not affect their health or energy levels.

These food "philosophies" may not work for everyone. This is one of the challenges of dieting; we all metabolize foods differently and our bodies have different needs that must be addressed for optimal health. There is a practice called Metabolic Typing. This helps you to assess which combination of foods is best for a particular person, as to their health and energy needs:

More Carbohydrates and less Fat and Protein

More Protein, a little Fat, and Less Carbohydrates

A balanced combination of Carbohydrates and Proteins with a little bit of Fat

As mentioned before, the average individual needs a balanced, high quality combination of both protein and carbohydrates with a little bit of fat; this assures an even amount of energy distribution throughout the day. From that point you can alter it accordingly to your energy requirements and even look into various metabolic typing programs or practitioners that specialize in that type of program. The challenge is that most people consume processed carbohydrates as their primary food source, hence the increase in obesity that we have seen escalate throughout the years. The average person does not fare well with these proportions; they need more protein and fat to help stabilize their energy without having to resort to caffeine. As for children they typically need more protein and quality fat in order to stabilize their energy. Especially with school-aged children, your goal is to keep them satiated between meals. If they get hungry during class they will lose focus and become easily distracted, here is where their need for protein and quality fats helps them to stay fuller and focused longer.

A large difference in nutritional philosophies lies in the USDA Food Plate:

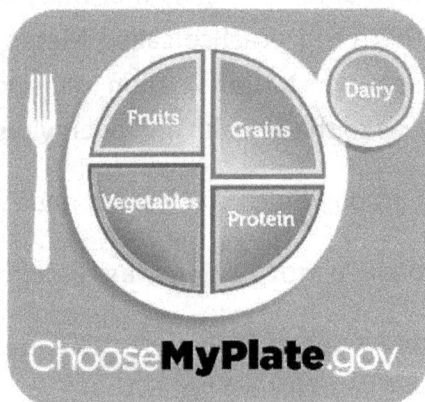

www.ChooseMyPlate.gov

Here you will notice how the proportions are more geared to a high carbohydrate food plan as opposed to a balanced one. Unfortunately, this is what a traditional dietician or nutritionist would prescribe as an eating template. Our philosophy stems from the nutritional density of foods and the understanding of how different foods impact our bodies. This helps us to provide our families with all of the nutritional needs for growth, brain development, and enhanced immune function.

This is where the Standard American Diet has been created, aka S.A.D., which relishes manufactured foods for a quick and easy meal with very little emphasis on fruits and vegetables. This is truly SAD; it has given rise to increased obesity, diabetes, high cholesterol, cancer, etc., etc., and leaves the body with very few nutrients for health. Blood sugar stays high and disease finds a home. Here is where you can clearly see how the food industry has been able to manipulate us into believing that they are looking out for our best interest. With the above Food Plate one could easily put in breakfast cereal with milk, sausage, juice, and potatoes, and theoretically hit almost all of the proportions right on. Unfortunately, the body needs nutrients and enzymes for optimal health, so with a Food Plate like this the body's only resolve is to struggle with health, both for ourselves and our children.

By using a more balanced approach to food proportions we can stabilize blood sugar, energy and health. The "Nutraterian" approach encourages a pyramid more like this one:

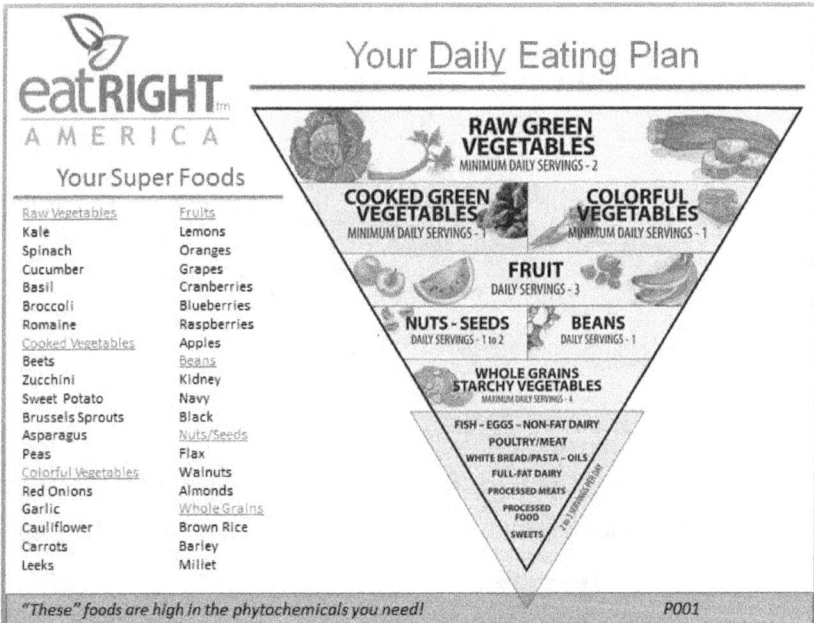

www.eatrightamerica.com

Eating for Daily Energy Requirements

Food is fuel, it is not comfort or socialization. A Ferrarri does not take in gasoline to hang out with other Ferraris, it takes in gasoline to take off like a rocket and show others its dust! Food is the exact same thing for us and our families, some foods empower us and others slow us down, the key is to choose the right ones with the activity of our day in mind. This will enable us to focus, stay stong, and maintain a lean body at all times. So here are a few examples:

a. Your child eats breakfast at 7 a.m. but won't have lunch until 12:00 p.m. You're not sure if they will get a snack in, so how do you choose the right food proportions? Ok, if you go the traditional route, you would have them have a bowl of cereal with milk and a glass of juice. All of these metabolize fast and act as a sugar, so they would probably find themselves looking around their classroom by 10 a.m., even a bit antsy, basically because they are starving and really don't realize it. On the other hand, if you made them a couple of eggs with a bit of fruit on the side, or better yet an avocado, you would have given them enough protein and fat to help prolong the breakdown of the calories so that they would stay fuller longer and make it through to lunchtime.

b. Another example of this is a salad. A basic salad with iceberg lettuce, tomato, and olive oil will last you a very short time. On the other hand, if you took that same salad, added more vegetables, kale, sunflower seeds, chicken, and olive oil that salad would keep you fuller for a longer period of time.

c. Now, let's say you are eating dinner and going right to bed. You are better off with a higher carbohydrate meal that can quickly metabolize so that nothing stays sitting in your system and gets stored as fat. So for this a vegetable salad or stir-fry would work best.

So What's the Next Step?

Food proportions are an important aspect of any food plan. When raising a family, you have a variety of energy levels that you are dealing with, and teaching each member of the family how to maximize those levels with the right food proportions is golden.

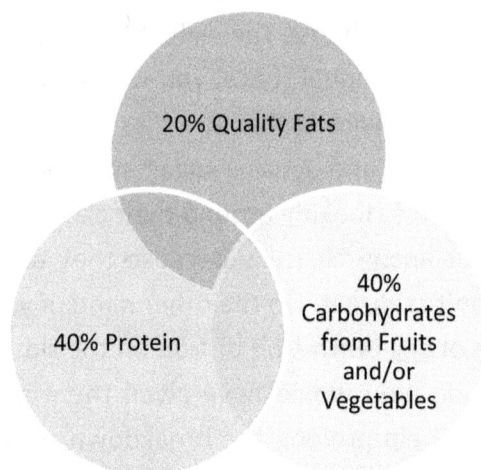

20% Quality Fats

40% Protein

40% Carbohydrates from Fruits and/or Vegetables

Here are a few clues to help you guide your family in choosing the right proportions for each meal and snack. As I mentioned earlier, we all metabolize foods differently. In other words, you may have one child who thrives on high protein and another who needs more carbohydrates, so here are your clues:

- If someone is famished before their next meal or snack, their proportion of protein was probably not enough in their previous meal
- If they are sleepy before a meal, the previous meal probably did not have enough carbohydrates and if they are sleepy right after a meal then their proportions of protein and fat may have been too high.

- If they are doing sports or had a very active day and seemed to crash at the end of the day, they probably didn't have sufficient fat in their meals and snacks
- And, of course, if the proportions were good but the symptoms still came up, they may be dehydrated and simply needing more water throughout the day.

How Can You Make a Change? I realize that some of you are already living a very healthy lifestyle while others are overwhelmed with each page in this book. Changing the food plan and lifestyle of a home is only going to be as challenging as you make it. Change comes best when handled one step at a time. You cannot expect to change the pallet of your family overnight, but you can start to instill a few changes each month until you reach your goal. Sometimes you may even have to mask some of the healthier options with a few unhealthy staples just so that you can get it into the house, and guess what... That is OK your goal is to make changes one step at a time and with all of the stress that we as parents have on a day-to-day basis, food should not be one of them.

On the same note it is important to teach your family about making the right food choices and have them begin to notice the change in energy, health or focus. The more you can encourage the positive feelings they are receiving from their new food choices the better.

Notes, Stuff to Remember, Things to Buy, etc.

Food Challenges

This section is included because I feel it is important for you, as a parent, to understand and become aware of a few of the challenges that could affect your family.

Physical Challenges

The following are physical challenges that would have an impact on a person's weight, health or general food plan. These are either hereditary or "symptoms of life", they can occur from childhood or start up during any stage of life. Some may go away, while others are there for the duration, it is all about making a commitment to make changes:

Food Allergies

A food allergy is a serious medical condition that triggers the immune system and affects millions of individuals. The job of the body's immune system is to identify and destroy germs (such as bacteria or viruses) that make you sick. A food allergy results when the immune system mistakenly targets a harmless food protein as an allergen, and a threat, and attacks it.

Unlike other types of food disorders, such as intolerances, food allergies are "IgE mediated". This means that your immune system produces abnormally large amounts of an antibody called immunoglobulin E—IgE for short. IgE antibodies fight the "enemy" food allergens by releasing histamine and other chemicals, which trigger the symptoms of an allergic reaction. These symptoms can be as mild as a rash or as "life threatening" as the inability to breathe or worse (anaphylaxis). Most food allergies can be recognized with a blood test from your physician, and once the allergens are identified and removed from a food plan, all symptoms will dissipate unless the allergen is introduced again.

Food Intolerances

Food intolerances or food sensitivity occurs when a person has difficulty digesting a particular food. This can lead to symptoms such as intestinal gas, abdominal pain, rashes, itchy skin, acne or even diarrhea. Food intolerances are sometimes confused with or mislabeled as a food allergy. Food intolerances involve the digestive system and can easily lead to severe weight gain. While the body is digesting foods, the particular intolerance triggers digestive distress, and as a defense mechanism the body will store whatever is combined with the intolerance as fat.

The easiest way to recognize food intolerances is by recording what you eat and how you feel from those foods in a food log or journal. The challenge arises when a dish has several ingredients; list them all, and with time the intolerant food will become clear. Another way of figuring out intolerances is through a blood test, typically performed by an alternative medicine practitioner (just

FYI, western medicine does not acknowledge food intolerances).
Food intolerances are not always permanent and many times
removing the food for 90 days or more will solve the intolerance
and the food will be able to be introduced again.

Diabetes

This is listed here because diabetes requires the reduction or
elimination of carbohydrates, especially those that break down as
a sugar. According to the Mayo Clinic, diabetes mellitus refers to a
group of diseases that affect how your body uses and breaks
down blood sugar (glucose). Glucose is vital to your health
because it's an important source of energy for the cells that make
up your muscles and tissues. It's also your brain's main source of
fuel.

If you have diabetes, no matter what type, it means you have too
much glucose in your blood, although the causes may differ. Too
much glucose can lead to serious health problems; therefore, you
don't want to add any additional sugar (carbohydrates) from foods.
Chronic diabetes conditions include type 1 diabetes and type 2
diabetes. There are also potentially reversible diabetes conditions,
which include pre-diabetes—when your blood sugar levels are
higher than normal but not high enough to be classified as
diabetes—and gestational diabetes, which occurs during pregnancy
but may resolve after the baby is born. No matter what type of
diabetes one has, it is important to minimize carbohydrates,
especially those that metabolize as a sugar such as sugar, flour,
dairy, and alcohol, and emphasizing lower glycemic fruits and
vegetables and more proteins and fats.

Psychological Challenges / Eating Disorders

"An eating disorder is an obsession with food and weight that harms a person's well-being", as stated by the American Psychology Association. Eating disorders seriously threaten physical and psychological health. The cause of eating disorders is unknown, but suggested causes link the psychological aspect of the disorder. Individuals may believe that they would be happier and more successful if they were thin, they have a need to be perfect and are consumed with the pressures that society places on people to be as lean as possible. They allow stress, over-commitment, and the need to feel "in control" to dictate their feelings about themselves. Most often, eating disorders are found in teenage girls, but they can also occur in teenage boys, women, and men. Treatment often includes medical intervention, counseling or therapy, and, in some cases, hospitalization.

Eating disorders are psychological disorder and typically stem out of the normal range of parenting. In other words, here is where a trained professional is advisable. Our children watch everything; sometimes we, as parents, don't recognize our own obsessions with weight loss and exercise. We may feel that they are mild but our child's interpretation takes it to the extreme and they begin to create their own definition of lean and muscular. So with this said, the following information is more "informational" so that you can identify any challenges arising in your family.

No one likes to think they are doing something wrong; it can become a tricky situation with a child, but as their parent you can find the right support and resolve the issues from the beginning. Remember, our job is to educate our children and provide them with the right foundation.

Medical and psychological complications associated with eating disorders include:	
Gastrointestinal /digestive irregularities	Sleep disorders
Cardiac arrhythmias - irregular heart beat	Excessively dry sky
Hypotension - low blood pressure	Low self-esteem
Hypothermia - cold intolerance	Depression, anger, anxiety
Dehydration	Low frustration tolerance
Amenorrhea	High need for approval

Anorexia is a condition in which a person is obsessed with being thin. Anorexics lose a lot of weight and are terrified of gaining weight. They don't want to eat and may constantly worry about how many calories they consume or how much fat is in their food. They may use diet pills, laxatives, and water pills to lose weight and may exercise too much.

The warning signs of anorexia include:	
Deliberate self-starvation with weight loss	Greater amounts of hair on the body or the face
Fear of gaining weight	Sensitivity to cold temperatures
Refusal to eat	Absent or irregular menstruation - Amenorrhea
Denial of hunger	Loss of scalp hair
Constant exercising	A self-perception of being fat when the person is really too thin

Bulimia is characterized by a person who eats a lot of food at one time (binging) and then throws up or uses laxatives to remove the food from the body (purging). Some bulimics may fast or over-exercise after binging to keep from gaining weight. Bulimics may use water pills, laxatives, and diet pills to "control" their weight and usually stash food and hide binging behavior.

The warning signs of bulimia include:	
Obsessive pursuit of thinness	Dental and gum disease
A bitter/sour halitosis - VERY bad breath	Gastrointestinal /digestive Irregularities
Unusual eating habits and behaviors	Dehydration
Absent or irregular menstruation – Amenorrhea	

- Preoccupation with food (binges on carbohydrates, high fluid intake, eats fast and in large bites, can't waste food, somewhat aware of calories).
- Complications associated with diuretic and laxative use such as bloating, diarrhea, constipation, fatigue, muscle cramps, and decreased bone density.

Binge Eating Disorder, also called compulsive overeating, is characterized by eating unusually large amounts of food and often feeling guilty or secretive. People with a binge eating disorder have a different relationship with food. At first food may provide sustenance or comfort, but eventually it may become the focus of guilt or distress. People with this condition eat large amounts of food quickly and feel completely out of control as they do it. It is different than occasionally eating too much in that there is a loss of control and a feeling that you cannot stop or control how much you are eating. It differs from anorexia and bulimia as people with binge eating disorder are usually overweight. The most common health risks are the same as those that accompany obesity. The causes are unknown, but many people who binge eat say that it is triggered by feelings of anger, sadness, boredom or anxiety. The warning signs of binge eating disorder include:

- A pattern of eating in response to emotional stress, such as family conflict, peer rejection, and poor academic performance.
- Feeling ashamed or disgusted by the amount of food eaten.
- Finding food containers hidden in the person's room or house.
- Possessing an increasingly irregular eating pattern, such as skipping meals, eating lots of junk food, and eating at unusual times (like late at night).

These are challenging issues when you are dealing with a family member. Just keep in mind that many times we, as the adults, are the ones that outwardly obsess about our appearance and our weight and this can have a huge effect on a family member's relationship with food. These disorders can have detrimental effects on the body and the health of an individual. You are placed in a very uncomfortable position, but your inspiration and guidance can save them from themselves. Their health and wellbeing is in your hands so reaching out to a trained professional, even if you are simply speculating, is your best course of action.

Behavior Modification

Behavior modification is simply the changing of behaviors or bad habits. This is probably the hardest aspect of health and weight management, but, at the same time, it is the most essential. Without change, anything you do to impact your health or weight is temporary. Most people will achieve their health and weight goals and go right back to the habits that made them unhealthy in the first place. Behavioral modifications and goal setting will help to create lifestyle changes for an everyday Food Plan.

This section is designed more for you, as the parent, than for your children. No matter how you look at it, you are their role model and how you view your health, weight, and wellbeing reflects how they will view theirs today, tomorrow, and for a lifetime. If you, or an older child, are challenged with weight, energy levels or health, the first place to start is with a Food Log. Writing out everything you eat each and every day, and documenting how you feel, can have a tremendous impact on the psychology of you and food. We have all been programed from childhood to think of food as a reward; it is a comfort and a host of other "warm and fuzzy" things... not! FOOD IS FUEL.

A good Food Log keeps track of the type of food eaten, when the food was eaten, the carbohydrate/sugar to protein ratio, how the body feels (gassy, bloated, energized, sleepy), and has a space to record behavior changes and exercise habits. This is meant as a motivational tool so the information used can be as detailed as you want, written in whatever manner that can help you or a family member recognize the areas that need change. (You can easily use the Food Log provided on P. 104)

Below is a list of additional behavior change ideas that you may want to use. The most important thing to remember is to only choose one or two changes at a time and to set a realistic plan of action to accomplish those changes. Habits won't change overnight; they say it takes 21 days to create a habit and at the same time it takes that much or sometimes longer to undo a habit. There are some experts who may not agree with the "21 day" example, but it makes a good visual and achievable timeline that may help. Draw out charts, create a reward system (without using food) or figure out just the right "thing" to be able to praise the progress and celebrate the changes that are made.

Things to remember:

Preplan your meals, including snacks	Remove foods that make you feel gassy or bloated
Eliminate tempting foods from your home	Remove your plate as soon as you've finished eating
Drink plenty of water before a meal	Minimize or eliminate processed foods
Share a menu item instead of eating it all yourself	Change to non-binging friends
Celebrate in a non-food, non-drink way	When stress takes over, have a cup of tea in a relaxed manner instead of a snack
Do not keep serving dishes on the table	Practice relaxation exercises
Use smaller plates, bowls, glasses, and serving spoons	Put leftovers away before you sit down to eat

Notes, Stuff to Remember, Things to Buy, etc.

The 4 Components of Foundational Health

As you coach your family with great foods and awesome nutrition, you also want to be the advocate for unstoppable health. Health is an amazing thing, but unfortunately there is no one thing that encompasses complete health. Only a balanced approach will lead to a foundation of great health and longevity. With this said, the primary factors that create a strong foundation for our health are the following:

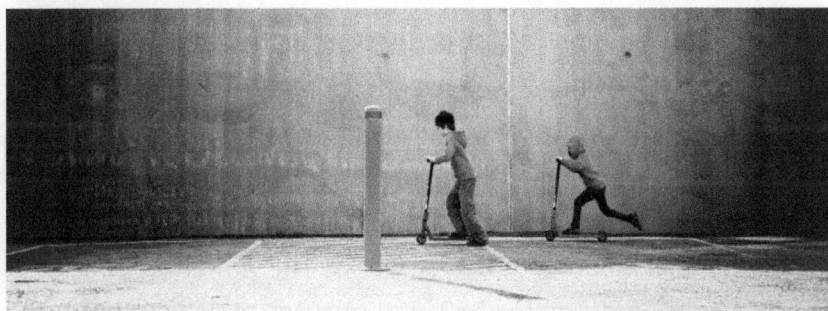

Exercise

Our bodies are designed to move, this enhances fluidity of movement, which brings about strength in the muscle and encourages elimination of toxins and fat. Every member of your family NEEDS to move! Running, jumping, lifting, playing, it all raises your heart rate and that is a good thing. A good exercise program should be comprised of cardiovascular/endurance type exercise, strength training, and flexibility. Think of it this way: cardiovascular conditioning encourages circulation, strength adds power to that circulation, and flexibility opens the body to receive all of the benefits of that circulation. Also, as your kids get older, movement will become an everyday occurrence. Once again, it is about creating the foundation of health so that they begin to live by it without being told.

There are hundreds of ways of enhancing one's fitness level, it is all about increasing your heart rate and breaking a sweat. So please don't think that the gym is the only place to go; the playground, the back yard, a trampoline, sports, and so much more can easily get the job done. With your family, it should all be about FUN!

A good combination of structured exercise and other FUN activities can provide a well-rounded program for most of the family! The old standby of performing 60 minutes of consecutive exercise has now changed to a "friendlier" approach; small bouts of exercise throughout the day are just as good. So if 10 minutes is all you have at the moment that works. The American College of Sports Medicine promotes 150–300 minutes of activity per week (150 minutes for a novice and 300 for the enthusiast), how you break it down is up to you.

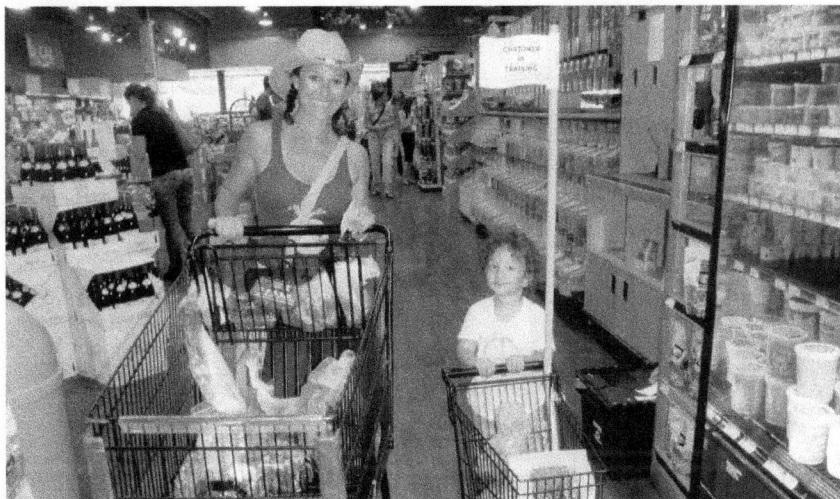

Nutrition

The right food choices can enhance your energy, recuperation, and so much more. As you have seen in the previous pages, nutrition has a large impact on our overall health and, once combined with the other three foundational components, can provide our bodies with a strong structure inside and out. The main thing is to educate your family so that they have a good understanding that not all calories are created equal; it's all about eating for the quality of our foods rather than the quantity!

"Always remember you are growing an adult from scratch, one bite at a time!"

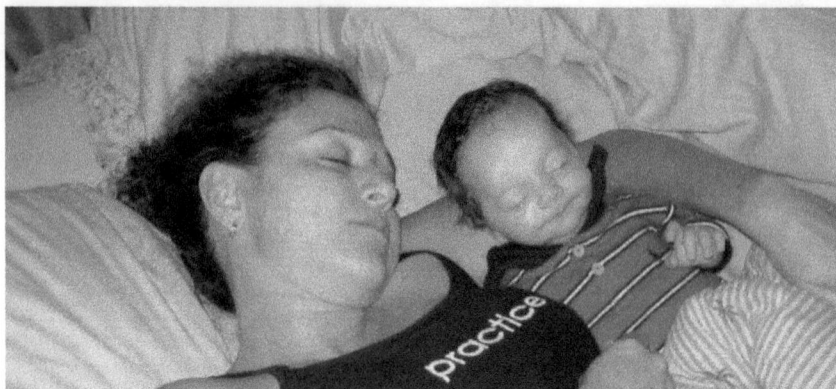

Sleep and Relaxation

Sleep and the ability to defuse and destress are a huge component of health. The average adult needs about 8 hours of sleep per night and the average child 10–12 hours per night. We are consumed with living our day, and many times our nights get shortened, but one must realize that what happens in our sleep can impact our day and our health. On the flip side, the ability to minimize stress or simply understand how to deal with it is just as important. The demands placed on a child from school, peers, and responsibilities can be overwhelming when they don't have the tools to learn how to let the pressures go. As you help to form their foundation, these are things that you can also help them to learn and grow with.

A lack of sleep is one of the number one things that can affect how we deal with daily stresses. Additionally, a lack of quality sleep can affect how we digest our foods, lose weight, focus, and grow. Ideally, our sleep patterns would mimic that of the sun and moon, realistically that will never happen! So our next best thing is to understand how our bodies function with rest and incorporate it as much as possible in order to reap the benefits. We have hundreds of hormones that have some major roles to play in the body, but for our purposes here we are going to stick to two of them:

Cortisol *(red line)*: A hormone manufactured in the adrenal glands. With normal sleep patterns, cortisol is regenerated during sleep and will naturally decline throughout the day and then lead into sleep. This hormone is directly involved in the metabolism of carbohydrates and influences our levels of glucose available for activity and energy throughout the day. It protects the body against stress but can be easily depleted with too much stress.

Serotonin *(blue line)*: A neurotransmitter that has a diverse multitude of functions but a regulator of mood, appetite, and sleep. With normal sleep patterns, serotonin kicks in at night, during sleep, and helps to repair and rejuvenate the muscles and the mind. Serotonin levels are affected by specific foods, nutrients and exercise—the more muscle one has the more serotonin is produced and the better we sleep.

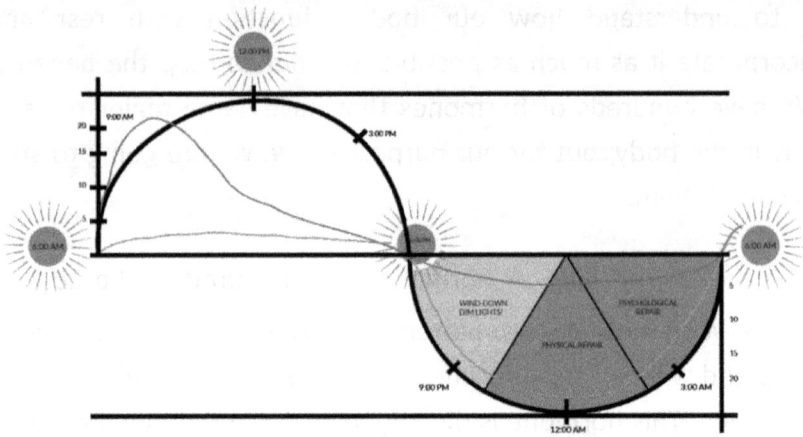

These are the two components that help to provide us with sufficient rest and recuperation and sufficient energy. Cortisol and serotonin cannot work at the same time. Cortisol is active during the day—light enhances it and helps to energize us; on the other hand serotonin kicks in with darkness and helps to bring us into a deep sleep. The key to optimal rest is to recognize that during the stage of serotonin, any light that comes to us, even if our eyes are closed, will awaken cortisol and disrupt our sleep. Once disrupted, or if disrupted throughout the night, this will then affect our physical and mental recuperation.

10:00 p.m. – 2:00 a.m. – Physical Repair: This is when our bodies recuperate from all of the physical activity it has received in the day. This is when our muscles develop, grow stronger, and repair any damage.

2:00 a.m. – 6:00 a.m. – Psychological Repair: This is when all of our thoughts, stresses, and emotions receive a time to disappear, forgive, or just chill, and our mind rejuvenates and grows.

So here it is in a nutshell – If someone constantly goes to bed late, their body will not repair appropriately and their physical gains will take forever. On the flip side, if they are constantly getting up way too early, their mind doesn't have a chance to truly relax, leaving them stressed during the day and leaving them with little energy to put their all into their studies and activities.

As crazy as this may seem, this is so closely interrelated to one's success both in life and in school. The body is well rested when we can wake up refreshed. If we are challenged to wake up then something has disrupted our sleep. Here are a few challenges to look for that can be easily changed to improve the quality of sleep for the entire family:

1. The room should be pitch dark. In other words, NO LED LIGHTS from video game consoles, TVs, stereos or anything else. I recommend using tape to place a small piece of cardboard over each of the little lights in a room.
2. The room should be COLDER than usual; a chill in the air induces better quality sleep.
3. Stop all electronics (cell phone, TV, tablet, computer, etc.) one hour before bed. Also, if used at night, be sure to set the display on night shift to remove the blue light from stimulating your cortisol.
4. Keep minimal electronics in the room, ideally all computers and cell phones should be plugged in a different room.

Additionally here are a few tricks to induce slumber:

1. Meditation or yoga before bedtime can help bring the body back to calm after a challenging day. Children of all

ages can benefit, and many schools have incorporated even a small sample of these into their curriculum, so take advantage of that and bring it into the home.

2. Sleepy teas – create a family ritual of an after dinner sleepy tea, like chamomile, valerian root or kava, to soothe everyone down for rest.

3. Reading a "paper" book in bed can also do the trick.

Sleep affects everything in our lives and many feel that they don't need that much sleep to survive. Well, that word "survive" is the key phrase. We should not feel satisfied with just "surviving", we need to live and live large.

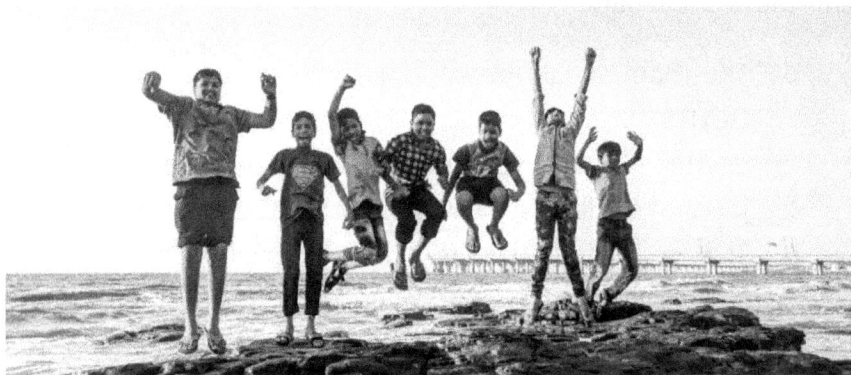

Happiness

Yes, life's enjoyment also plays a pivotal role in our health—who knew? Making it a priority to enjoy as much as you can in your day-to-day has a huge impact when combined with the other four components. Without happiness we cannot motivate and encourage others to be their very best, we lose drive and enthusiasm, resulting in sluggishness and lethargy. Life is meant to be enjoyed and personal satisfaction and gain come from goals and aspirations that drive us to be our very best. Age has no limit here; this foundation that we are building for the "future adults" we are developing, needs fun and laughter as the high of life. As a parent, you are the inspirational source for your family, and friends for that matter; what you do and say can affect someone's day, month or year, so it's not just about their happiness, it's also about your own happiness and how that translates to those around you!

We Only Live Once!

Here are a few things to consider that Life Coach Barry Gotlied shared one day:

- ♠ Avoid the news, say, "*No,*" to television, radio, and negative publications
- ♠ Don't condemn, criticize or complain ... become a solution finder and encourage your children to do the same
- ♠ Get rid of the "*Negatrons*" in your life – surround yourself with positive people
- ♠ Look for and share stories about positive people and events, share them with your family and friends
- ♠ Have an attitude of gratitude. Share the things you are grateful for and have your family do the same
- ♠ Read something inspirational, educational or spiritual each day
- ♠ Replace your limiting beliefs and fears with new, positive, empowering beliefs
- ♠ Take ownership of your life, seize the moment!

You want to teach your family to focus on the positive and minimize the negative, making it a priority to laugh each and every day. Surround yourself with and encourage your kids to choose friends who inspire and encourage them to be their very best. It's like the saying goes, "If you want to lose weight, eat lunch with your skinny friends." So if you want to increase your happiness, hang out with your "happy friends" and make yourself one of those" happy" people that others love to be with.

Everything in your life is your choice, you have the choice to listen, absorb or walk away. Responsibility for one's life is one of the hardest concepts to grasp, not because we don't understand it but because it's much easier to blame others for our challenges. Here's where parenting has to take it up a notch, we want to give our children the tools to become amazing adults, and although this has little to do with nutrition and exercise, it is still an integral part of health.

Here's a little exercise for you to do, but it is a good one to share with your kids as well:

Take a moment and consciously take note of the things you tend to blame others for. Now choose one of those things and think about another solution if you could not blame anyone for it (i.e. "I gain weight because my husband wants to drink wine every night." You have the choice to drink wine or not, so the weight gain is not his fault it is yours. "Every time I walk to class this kid tries to trip me." Maybe you simply need to say, "Hi," maybe they just want your attention) This makes things a bit harder, some mental cleansing may need to happen, but in the long run it will make you a happier and healthier person for yourself and for those around you.

It's All a Balancing Act

Balance these 4 components and you have maximized the health of you and your family for life! Putting too much emphasis in one area will throw your system off, no matter how "healthy" that area of your life is. It is all about utilizing the 4 components to work and thrive together so that your health and the health of your family is strong, energizing, and empowering!

"Parenting is challenging no matter how you look at it. Creating a healthy environment that encourages healthy habits will be ingrained in their DNA for years to come. They may sway off the wagon here and there, but their health foundation will always bring them back!"

SuperPower Shut-Eye Evaluator

Sleep can be our friend or our worst enemy. It is what helps us recuperate both physically and mentally from the day before. Without providing the proper recuperation we can often find ourselves drowsy, with a lack of concentration and unmotivated to reach our goals. We can also find that our recovery period from school, exercise, or our day is nonexistent and that our bodies remain tired, sore or even injured.

Please answer the following questions to see where you stand on proper rest and relaxation:

1. What time do you go to bed at night?_____

2. What time do you wake up?_____

3. What time do you typically work out?_____

4. How many days per week?_____

5. When you wake up, do you feel rested or groggy?_____

6. How long does it usually take you to fall asleep?
    a. 0–5 minutes
    b. 5–15 minutes
    c. 15–30 minutes
    d. More than 30 minutes

7. On average, how many times do you wake up during the night (circle the correct response)?
   None   1   2   3   4   5   6 or more

8. Why do you wake up during the night?
    a. nature calls
    b. dreams or nightmares
    c. external noise
    d. other:

Now, here's your chance to really see what's going on. Review the following:

10:00 p.m. – 2:00 a.m. – **Physical Repair**: This is when our bodies recuperate from all of the physical activity they have received in the day. This is when our muscles develop, grow stronger, and repair any damage. So my question to you is, "Are you providing uninterrupted sleep during this time?" If not, is there something that you can change to make it better?

2:00 a.m. – 6:00 a.m. – **Psychological Repair**: This is when all of our thoughts, things we have learned, stresses, and emotions receive time to disappear or grow, forgive or just chill and our mind gets to rejuvenate from it all. So again I ask, "Are you providing uninterrupted sleep during this time?" If not, is there something that you can change to make it better?

What are two things you can do to maximize your recovery through sleep?

1. _____

_____

2. _____

_____

SuperPower STRESS Check

Are you managing your stress in a healthy, effective manner? Answer the following questions so that we can make sure that you are on the right track. Add the total number of YES's and use the information at the bottom of the page to interpret your score.

1. Sometimes I am overwhelmed with the amount of things I need to get done in a day.
2. My head pounds for no reason at all, more than most.
3. I can get so carried away with "stuff" that I forget to eat.
4. I can go from grumpy to nice in a blink of an eye.
5. I often use food, drugs, alcohol or caffeine to create my "stress free" ahh moment.
6. By the end of the day I am exhausted, tired, and "DONE"!
7. I often feel like a bloated stomach is my norm.
8. If someone could look inside my head they would be exhausted from everything that is running around at once.
9. Sometimes I feel the pitter patter of ... my heart racing and wanting to pound out of my chest.
10. Who needs sleep? I often spend the evening trying to get to sleep or staring at the shadows on the ceiling.
11. I worry a lot about tomorrow in hopes that it gives me a better today.
12. Bah humbug, who needs purpose or fulfillment? I'm like this most of the time and I'm OK.
13. I keep a far distance from my friends and family, some might call it withdrawal, I just call it avoidance!
14. If I need to focus and concentrate on a normal basis, I hire someone.
15. I sometimes criticize myself because I know everyone else is criticizing me too.

16. If I can't control it, somehow it controls me.
17. Life can be fun; I just don't have the time to enjoy it right now.
18. I can catch a cold just from getting sneezed on.
19. Food is my friend and my stress buddy.
20. Who is on edge? I'm just wired differently than you.

Now, let's see how you did.
Remember this is just a general analysis and it should be a good eye-opener to keep you on the right path of health.

0–7 MILD – Awesome! If you answered YES to seven or fewer items then your stress is MILD and manageable. In other words, you are coping very well and can recover from stress in a healthy manner. Keep up the good work, and continue finding more ways to relax and enjoy yourself!

8–13 MODERATE – How do you feel? If you answered YES to 8–13 items then your stress is MODERATE. At this point you are not recovering from stress as best as you can and still holding on to some of it. Your body and mind are giving you subtle hints that they are not happy and need some relaxation. Re-evaluate your priorities and recognize when the stress is there and take action to make it go away!

14–20 SEVERE – Oh No! If you answered YES to 14–20 items then your stress is SEVERE. This means that stress is making an impact on your health, happiness, and longevity. Your ability to cope and recover from day-to-day stresses is functioning at the bare minimum and you need to act on it! You are not functioning to your peak performance level and you are hampering your health. It's time to really set your priorities straight, create a good relaxation program and start placing your needs first. If stress has brought you to this point it is also time to call in the cavalry—visit your family physician and make a plan of action to set your health on the path it deserves.

Family Health Cheat Sheet

Health has so many definitions but no matter how you look at it, it is the foundation for our health, energy, and stamina until death. Motherhood comes with its own set of challenges but one of our primary jobs is to raise healthy kids inside and out. Before you get all crazy with the details, simply realize that this is so much more than forcing broccoli as a side dish (hopefully you have learned this here already). This is about teaching habits that will take a toddler to elementary school, through high school, and into college, and then all the way to business woman or man extraordinaire!

As a means of keeping this as simple as possible, let's take each facet of life and discuss the habits that will be the stepping stones to the next phase.

Toddlers

This is a time when flavors are starting to develop and where the art of cooking and manipulating flavors can be so powerful. Here is where you hide some of the most nutritious of items just to create combinations that are tasty enough to the pickiest of eaters, yet bringing in a host of nutrition with each bite. Getting your kids involved in the kitchen is paramount at this stage. I realize it can be a messy endeavor, but the lessons of flavors and tasting will be invaluable and will make your life easier as they grow and become more boisterous with their thoughts and feelings. Simple things like marinara sauce, ground beef, smoothies, and even pancakes can hide so much more than you can imagine. Your food processor should be your best friend in the kitchen. Also, this is the time to start talking about proteins and get them to know what a protein is, granted it won't happen overnight but you can start laying down the ground work.

Great health also incorporates activity, playing and running should be a main staple of exercise. Making sure they get their movement in before TV or electronics makes a great habit for years to come. I hate to say it but toddlers are like dogs, they need to be run to get all of their energy out in a healthy productive manner. And If you play your cards right, you should be getting in on some of that, the bonding is awesome and the calories burned are even better!

Elementary School Age

These tikes have their opinions, but you hold the keys to the kitchen. Your children will not starve, and I say this to you with love. Many kids will demand a different dish and it is up to you to stay strong and create enough variety in the food offerings of a meal. There should be no thought of making something else simply to get them to eat. If you have already been exposing your children to the kitchen you should have a good eater, if you have not, it is time to get them to make something. The more exposure they have, the more they will be open to tasting and trying new things. It is time to make sure they incorporate a fruit or a vegetable with every meal and snack. They will gravitate towards the processed food choices if you let them, but let that happen at a friend's house and not at yours. Your home needs to be the forefront of health. In my home we have a "4 taste rule"; foods need to be tasted on 4 different occasions before it can be deemed evil.

As for the fitness side of thing, this is a time for sports or outdoor play for hours on end. Everything works better with some activity, your brain, your energy, and your attitude. Encouraging activity before TV and electronics sets the stage for habits when they are older.

High School

Ok my friends this is a time where your kids need to be making breakfast for YOU. By now they should be able to cook eggs and follow a basic recipe, you are training them to function completely on their own and it is time they kick in. They should completely understand food choices and how their energy is impacted by the wrong choices, how the right combination of proteins, fats, and carbohydrates can empower them or drain them. They are old enough to buy their own snacks so this is where the previous years of coaching will show its true colors.

As for fitness, you would hope that they would gravitate to a sport in their elementary years. Keeping them in an organized sport is so much easier at this point then trying to think of what they can do to stay in shape. For those in organized sports you should be good to go, on the other hand for those who have no plan, this is a great time for you to see about taking a class or activity together. Your about to lose them to college so if you can create a bonding time, relish it. If not simply encourage them to do something with a group of friends. Movement needs to be a part of their day to day; these are the habits that will translate to college and beyond. Also, keep in mind that muscle has memory, so even if they place their fitness on hold during some of their college years, they will have a fit foundation and it will be so much easier to become fit once it is said and done.

College and Beyond

Your coaching will come full circle at this point. You are sending your young ones off into the world with hopes they make the right choices and that you have instilled the right habits to carry them through. Think of it this way, do you want to send out an overweight, lazy, junk food junky into the world or would you prefer a well-nourished, active, adult who can cook great meals and is a snob for good nutrition.?

Now we all have our challenging cases, but with love and persistence keeping an active lifestyle and choosing the right food choices can become the day to day life of your entire family, it is all in how you present it, you got this!

"Remember, your child will not starve. Many a time has my daughter told me she does not like what I made and won't eat it. I simply tell her that is what there is, and if she doesn't want to eat it she will...starve. OK, some of you may think this is harsh but wait for it... 15-20 minutes later she comes back telling me she is ready to eat her dinner. Like I said, they will not starve!"

Notes, Stuff to Remember, Things to Buy, etc.

Creating Your Customized Livet®

N ow, with everything you have learned thus far, it's time to put it together in a usable and powerful Family Food Plan. A Livet® is a "food plan for living". Think about it, a traditional "diet" emphasizes "die", it's about ending the way you eat, torturing yourself by eating things you don't like, to lose a few pounds and then gain them back or to pick up your energy and then crash and lose focus towards the middle of your day. As a parent it is up to you to empower your family members with the knowledge to make wise choices for their health and activity throughout the day. So with this said, here is your template to help you set a food plan into motion that you and your family can thrive on. Get the family involved; create comradery and competition, whatever works to make this a fun learning activity.

Tools Needed: 3 different colored highlighters (feel free to add more highlighters to show water, caffeine or anything else you want to showcase)

STEP 1 – Have everyone write out everything they eat and drink for 5–10 days, including a weekend. Make sure to encourage them to be as detailed as possible, the more details the easier it is to guide them. Also, have them give you a list of their top ten favorite foods. For most it is easier to get a notebook and simply log in the foods and drink right after they eat them.

STEP 2 – Take a PINK highlighter and highlight everything that is sugar, flour, dairy or alcohol (and I do hope the alcohol is strictly for the adults ☺)

STEP 3 – Take the GREEN <u>highlighter</u> and highlight fruits and vegetables

STEP 4 – Take the YELLOW highlighter and highlight all protein (keeping in mind that dairy products do not provide sufficient protein and break down as a sugar so they would be PINK)

**Be sure to keep all Food Logs that have been highlighted, this will create a wonderful tracking system where you will easily be able to see how the changes have affected the plan. (Notice in the sample below how the green and yellow highlights are increased and the pink is decreased in the "ideal" scenario)

Here is a sample Adult and Child plan

Traditional Adult	Ideal Adult	Traditional Child	Ideal Child
9 a.m. Coffee with Cream and Sugar, Toast with Jam, slice of Watermelon 11 a.m. Bagel and Cream Cheese, Water 1:30 p.m. Sandwich with Turkey, Lettuce, Tomato, and Mayo. Chips, Ice Tea with Sugar 3 p.m. Coffee with Cream and Sugar, and 2 Chocolate Chip Cookies 8 p.m. Grilled Chicken with Small Salad, Bread, and Apple Pie and 2 Glasses of Wine	AM: 2 Glasses of Water Breakfast: Veggie Omelet with sliced Cantaloupe and a cup of Green Tea 2 Glasses of Water Snack: Apple with Almond Butter 2 Glasses of Water Lunch: Mixed Vegetable Salad with Chicken and Olive Oil 2 Glasses of Water Snack: Hummus and Carrots 2 Glasses of Water Dinner: Grilled Salmon with Asparagus Herbal Tea	7 a.m. Cereal with Milk and a glass of Juice 11 a.m. snack of Cheerios 1:30 p.m. Mac and Cheese with a glass of Milk 3 p.m. A handful of Goldfish and 2 Chocolate Chip Cookies with a glass of Juice 8 p.m. Grilled Chicken with Broccoli and Cheese and a glass of water	AM: 1 Glass of Water Breakfast: 2 Eggs with Sliced Cantaloupe and a glass of Water Snack: Apple with Almond Butter 1 Glasses of Water Lunch: Beans and Rice with Avocado on the side 1 Glasses of Water Snack: Hummus and Carrots 2 Glasses of Water Dinner: Grilled Salmon with roasted Sweet Potato

Your goal is to change the following:
1. Increase the water intake to a minimum of 8 glasses (6 or more for kids) and 2 more for anything caffeinated or alcoholic (the kids shouldn't have these ☺)
2. Every meal and snack should have an equal amount of protein and carbohydrates (preferably from fruits and vegetables)
3. Make sure that every meal and snack includes a fruit, vegetable or raw nuts or seeds
4. Allow zero to one sugar, flour, dairy or alcohol item per meal – with the hopes of taking it down further to only 2 per day

Ideal Meal /Snack layout for the
Average Person of any Age:
Protein + Carbohydrate + A Little Fat

With the above plan, you want to create an awareness of all of the sugars they are taking in. Remember these can cause any of the following:

✓ Obesity
✓ Lethargy
✓ Hyperactivity
✓ Distraction and Feeling Unfocused
✓ Acne and Skin Irritations

- ✓ High Cholesterol
- ✓ High Blood Sugar
- ✓ Joint Pain
- ✓ Low Immune Function
- ✓ And a host of other conditions and health related issues

This foundation that I keep talking about is the foundation of health for your youngest child all the way until they turn 50, who knew we had such power? You are creating the framework for all of their habits, as they relate to their health, that they will continue to follow throughout their life. The next page includes a blank Food Log that you can use with all of your family members. Make copies of it and create a bit of competition as everyone highlights their foods and creates their own plan to make changes. Many times putting the little ones in charge of the changes for the adults is a great way to instill these good habits into their day-to-day thinking.

Picky Eaters

I realize that many of the food challenges in the home have to deal with a picky eater at times or sometimes it's just written in the stars for that day. Either way, here's a few things to keep in mind:

1. It takes 4 times to truly decide if you love or hate a food. Make a deal with your children that they have to taste something at 4 different sittings before giving you the big old NO.

2. Get creative, your food processor can be your friend and hiding veggies or fruit in all sorts of recipes can be a good thing. Start with this and once they hit 6 or 7 years of age,

get them into the kitchen to help out and see the ingredients that have been going into their favorite dishes. Their opinion of some of those gross foods may change.

3. Work on getting a clear understanding of the flavors they like. Is it sweet, salty, spicy, etc.? Use this to help formulate some new recipes to get them trying a few new things.

4. For hard core picky eaters, simply add in something new once a month at the beginning. Use that same food once a week so you get in the 4 tastes in and see how that goes.

5. Get your kids into the kitchen at least once a month (although every week would be amazing). Let them get dirty and teach them about manipulating flavors in recipes and tasting while cooking. These are invaluable lessons. Most children don't know that you can manipulate or change the flavor of a recipe. Because of this they simply say NO to a particular food or dish. Wouldn't it be better if they could verbalize that it needs more salt, or needs to be sweeter? This can be a game changer for many households.

DAYS	Breakfast	Snacks	Lunch	Snacks	Dinner	Anything Additional
Monday						
Tuesday						
Wednesday						
Thursday						
Friday						
Saturday						
Sunday						

Family Nutrition Food Log

Once you have gathered all of the information from the food log and highlighted everything clearly, it makes it much easier to see the areas that need improvement and areas that have improved; together the family can formulate a plan of action to guide the group in a direction of health. The primary thing to keep in mind is that drastic changes never seem to work. The following is a typical progression that can be used:

1. Highlight the current food log and create a family discussion about the direction to take with their food plans
2. The first change should be to increase water throughout the day
3. Next, aim to increase protein with each meal and snack
4. Then work on increasing fruits and vegetables with more emphasis on vegetables
5. At the one-month mark, have the family make a new food log and repeat all of the steps above

Remember, these should be small, subtle changes. With this kind of a food plan there is no need to focus on calories. By removing the processed foods and the sugars the calories will naturally go down. Also, by increasing the protein with a small amount of fat, the body will feel fuller for a longer period of time. With the alterations in food proportions and the increase in nutrients from more vegetables and fruits, you will find that your family is eating smaller amounts of food yet feeling satisfied.

Special Considerations for the Ultimate Food Plan

1. Consider altering the amount of protein depending on when the next meal will come into play. An example of this is someone who has breakfast at 6 a.m. but won't have lunch until 1 p.m. with little chance of a snack. With this amount of time in between meals they should include some extra protein and fat so that they can stay fuller for a longer period of time. This is typical with a school-aged child who is dependent on a specific lunchtime at school.

2. Make provisions for the "Activity of Your Day". For those who have a very active day with workouts, running around, sports, etc. be sure to include more calories with an extra snack or two. On the other hand, if it is one of those lazy days on the couch then few calories are necessary and choosing foods that metabolize and break down easily are best (i.e. fruits and vegetables).

3. If fruits and vegetables have been the challenge of a lifetime for your family, try introducing a smoothie. Here's a great way to get in the veggies you need while using fruit to mask the taste. (See the recipes at the end of this manual)

4. Remember, if someone is on medications and special considerations from their physician be sure to collaborate with their health care provider to make the right choices in their food plan.

5. Every meal and snack consumed should leave the person feeling SATISFIED but not full. The idea is that by the next meal or snack they START to feel hungry, eat again towards satisfaction, and continue on from there.

6. Most food challenges come from eating for emotional or social support. It is important to recognize these moments and proceed accordingly. A good example of this is having a relaxation ritual already in place. What this means is to have something "you do" when stressed, exhausted, or upset — drink a cup of tea, take a walk, meditate, etc. On the flip side, if you know you are attending a party with tons of rich, creamy foods DONT GET THERE HUNGRY! Eat a meal or snack high in protein and fat so that, when you are in that situation, you feel content just tasting certain foods as opposed to eating everything in sight. This also applies to kids' birthday parties — load your kids up on protein and fat before they go to the party, this way they are not starving and will simply nibble on the treats.

7. Depriving someone of the foods they "love" will delay the success of any good nutritional program. This is about empowering your family with knowledge so that they make better choices and create substitutions because of the results, how they feel or how they are going to feel.

Hunger vs. Fullness

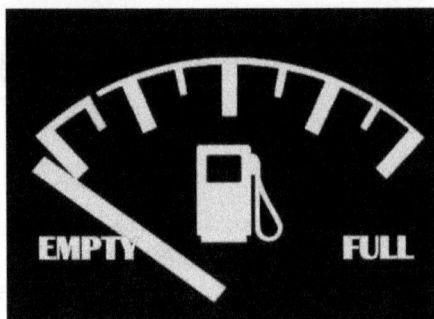

As I have mentioned before, the foods we give our children create their foundation, but with this there are other things that are important to teach as well. This may sound silly, but teaching our children about when they should eat, what they should eat, and when to stop eating all goes hand in hand.

There is so little said about this area, but it is one of the thresholds to health. This is our first response to make us aware that we may need food. Hunger does not mean starvation, hunger is the sensation that "we need food"; the question here is do we need food or do we need something else?

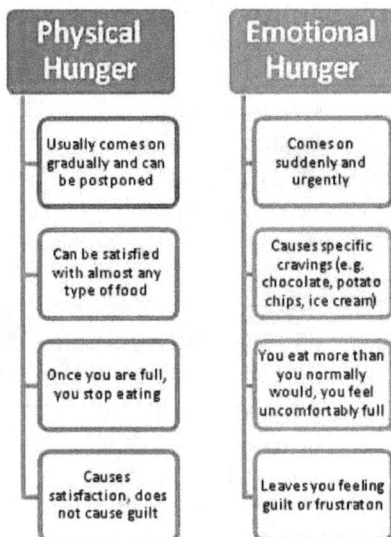

Physical Hunger	Emotional Hunger
Usually comes on gradually and can be postponed	Comes on suddenly and urgently
Can be satisfied with almost any type of food	Causes specific cravings (e.g. chocolate, potato chips, ice cream)
Once you are full, you stop eating	You eat more than you normally would, you feel uncomfortably full
Causes satisfaction, does not cause guilt	Leaves you feeling guilt or frustration

Physical Hunger is when you really need to eat and your body is completely set for the digestion and assimilation of food. This provides the body with a more positive response; you are content with natural foods. Genuine hunger symptoms include some of the following: Stomach feels empty; you're lightheaded and shaky.

Emotional Hunger is more of an appetite; it is how good food looks and smells, it is the enjoyment we get from food or the need for food because of the way we feel. These sensations create more of a negative effect on the mind and body. You may crave a specific food or feeling that you get from a specific food. Some of these symptoms include: Craving something specific, knowing you'll feel better if you eat something, and eating for no reason at all. Keep in mind that these are more LEARNED behaviors. As the parent these are things we want to be aware of, and we want to be able to teach our family how to handle situations differently as opposed to gravitating toward food when physical hunger is not the issue.

So now that you understand Hunger, how do you breakdown "Fullness"?

The key here is to teach your family to eat to feel "satisfied" and not "full". You want to eat somewhere between a 4 and a 5.

The Hunger Scale

1	2	3	4	5	6	7	8	9	10
Starving and feeling weak/dizzy.	Very hungry, irritable, low energy, large amounts of stomach growling.	Pretty hungry, stomach is beginning to growl.	Beginning to feel hungry.	Satisfied, niether hungry nor full.	Slightly full/ pleasantly full.	Slightly uncomfortable.	Feeling Stuffed.	Very uncomfortable, stomach aches.	So full you feel sick.

Notes, Stuff to Remember, Things to Buy, etc.

The Kitchen...

N ow let's set you up with some great recipes and food prep to get your kitchen moving in the right direction. Your first course of action is to prepare your kitchen and pantry for success; believe it or not, your family's health starts here.

Family Pantry Basics

Your pantry is the center of everything health and nutrition for your family, it is the basis of all recipes and all food plans. A well-stocked pantry will keep your family's food plan healthy and make sure that you have what you need for a well-designed meal, even when the pantry is at its emptiest!

The list below is designed simply as a guide, only you know what works best for you and the family. This list provides the basis of healthy cooking. Healthy cooking can be flavorful and easy. Be sure to choose organic when possible and read all ingredient lists—remember, if you can't pronounce it and don't know what it is ... don't eat it!

Basics

- Celtic or Himalayan Sea Salt – Fine and Coarse
- Black Peppercorns
- Extra Virgin Olive Oil – this one is for cooking
- Cold Pressed Olive Oil – this one is for salads or uncooked items
- Cold Pressed Coconut Oil – this one is for hundreds of things!
- Apple Cider Vinegar (with the mother – if you don't know what this is, don't worry; the label will tell you)
- Red Wine Vinegar
- Balsamic or Sherry Vinegar
- Rice Vinegar (unseasoned)

Sweeteners

- Dates
- Coconut Sugar
- Maple Syrup
- Raw Honey
- Stevia Leaf – make the tea, store it and pour as your sweetener
- Organic Unsweetened Apple Sauce

Grains

- Basmati or Jasmine Rice
- Red or Black Rice
- Wild Rice
- Quinoa
- Organic Popcorn Kernels
- Organic Rolled Oats

Fruits and Nuts

- Dried Fruit: Mulberries, Golden Berries, Goji Berries
- Raw Seeds: Sunflower, Flax, Pumpkin, Chia, Sesame or Hemp
- Raw Nuts: Almonds, Cashews, Walnuts, Pecans, Pine Nuts, Pistachios
- Raw Nut Butters: Almond, Cashew, Pecan

Packaged Goods

- Organic Chicken, Vegetable, or Bone Broth
- Beans: Cannellini, Navy, Chickpeas or Black
- Lentils
- Olives or Capers
- Diced or Roasted Tomatoes
- Tomato Paste
- Tomato Sauce
- Sun-dried Tomatoes
- Roasted Red Peppers
- Spicy Mustard

Fresh or Dried Herbs and Spices

– Keep in mind that fresh is always best, but the dried ones are great for backup. Dried herbs are best kept for 1 yr.

- Bay leaves
- Cayenne Pepper
- Chili Powder
- Crushed Red Pepper
- Curry Powder
- Fennel or Dill Seed
- Granulated Garlic
- Ground Cinnamon
- Ground Cloves
- Ground Cumin
- Ground Ginger
- Ground Coriander
- Turmeric
- Vanilla Extract
- Oregano
- Basil
- Parsley
- Paprika
- Rosemary
- Thyme
- Whole Nutmeg

Fresh Produce should be seasonal, local, and organic

when possible. Here are some wonderful resources to find yours:

- http://www.epicurious.com/articlesguides/seasonalcookin g/farmtotable/seasonalingredientmap
- http://www.micronutrients.com/wp-content/uploads/2015/07/ANDI-chart.pdf

But for the main staples of the home here are my top picks:

- Onions
- Garlic
- Avocados
- Carrots
- Celery
- Tomatoes
- Broccoli
- Bell Peppers
- Kale, Spinach or Collard Greens
- Lettuce: Romaine, Boston or Mixed Greens
- Cilantro
- Gingerroot
- Potatoes: Sweet or Purple
- Lemons
- Apples
- Berries
- Bananas

Freezer – *Remember that the freezer is a good place for backups and more. The following is a list of things that can be frozen without damaging the food.*

- All Raw Nuts can be frozen to preserve shelf life
- If Fruit is getting a bit soft, remember to freeze it for smoothies—you can either puree the fruit and freeze in an ice tray then store in an airtight container or chop and store in an airtight container

- Rice, Grains, and any form of Flour sometimes produce little bugs—by freezing these first you diminish the possibility of the bugs coming to life
- Frozen Peas, Broccoli and Berries are always good backups to have

Shelf Life 101.5

In our efforts to maintain a healthy kitchen we become possessive over all of the fad items, unused spices, and so much more that we can't manage to part with. The bottom line is that all foods provide us with the best nutrition when they are FRESH. But for the sake of convenience there are numerous items available that have a longer shelf life as long as we recognize what the "shelf life" looks like. Your goal is to steer clear of most preservatives and choose foods with minimal preservation techniques. Here are some of the top food categories and a few recommended storage techniques to assure quality and freshness:

Freezer and Refrigerator Cleanup

Think of it this way, the refrigerator is for the week, the freezer is backup and specific storage. The freezer should be that place where you have just enough to create a masterpiece meal when the fridge runs bare; then, when you go to the store, you can replace it all. For most of us, when the refrigerator runs empty, we tend to gravitate to eat anything in sight—good or bad. On that same note, the healthier the choices we begin to make the fewer processed foods we eat and the "cleaner" all of our choices are ... the emptier the fridge will be at the end of the week. For this reason a good refrigerator to freezer ratio makes an ideal situation for most. As for your fruits and veggies, creating good storage practices can enhance their shelf life a substantial amount. A good reference is *Dr. Richter's Fresh Produce Guide* by Henry Richter, he teaches you the ideal techniques for washing, storing, and taking care of your produce so they last.

Here's a timetable as a guide, remember that storage practices count so "how" you store it can affect how long it keeps for:

Food Item	Freezer time	Refrigerator Time
Baked Goods	3 months	1 week
Butter	1 year	1-2 weeks
Chicken – Raw	9 months	1-2 days
Condiments	very few will freeze	up to 1 year
Fish – Raw	6 months	1-2 days
Fruit Juices	1 year	2-3 days

Fruits	8 months – not optimal for all	up to 1 week, but some last longer
Ice Cream – Dairy	2 months	n/a
Ice Cream – Non-Dairy	6 months	n/a
Meats – Raw	9 months	1-2 days
Nuts	1 year	6 months
Shell Fish – Raw	1 year	1-2 days
Soups and Stews	3 months	4 days
Vegetables	8 months	Up to 1 week, but some can last longer

Pantry Cleanup

The pantry, or dry storage, is where most of our processed and manufactured items are stored along with our spices, baking ingredients, canned goods, and a few other things. Most of us take for granted that these items have unlimited shelf life; well, they don't and much, if any, of their nutritional value will deplete with time. Not to mention the amount of preservatives added in to preserve most of the manufactured foods. This is the area where you only want to store those things that will be readily used; it's best to continue to replenish in this area as keeping things longer than a year provides little if any health benefits.

"Keep in mind that nutrients die off with time"

Food Item	Shelf Life
Baking Mixes	9 months
Baking Powder	18 months
Baking Soda	2 years
Canned Fish	1 year
Canned Fruit or Vegetables	1 year
Crackers	3 months
Dried Fruit	6 months

Flour (all types)	1 year, but best in refrigerator or freezer
Honey and Syrups	1 year
Nuts	6 months
Pasta	1 year
Oils – Cold Pressed	1 year Or less (some become rancid)
Rice	1 year
Spices	Whole – 1-2 years / Ground – 6 months
Tea	1 year

You now have all of the tools to create your ultimate pantry. Make this fun and turn it into a family learning event—Your Yearly Pantry Clean Out! It's easier than you think. It's all about "Getting Started"; make a plan and your pantry will always be fresh and nutritious! Here are a few of my favorite tips to get you going:

🍃 Get the entire family involved. Review all of the ingredients in everything. If something contains high fructose corn syrup, preservatives or an ingredient that you can't pronounce and have no idea what it is, GET RID OF IT!

- Anything that is expired has GOT TO GO.
- Don't feel limited to the pantry, this clean out should also include the refrigerator and freezer.
- Get the family to help with re-organizing the pantry and refrigerator. Ideally everyone should be able to easily reach for their snacks and meal options. So for the little ones, be sure they have a reachable area to choose their favorite healthy bites from. One the same note, those items that are rarely used should be out of reach. I like to use baskets so that I can easily label what I have and place it towards the back or on a high shelf.
- And the hardest part of all is getting rid of this stuff! I know you spent good money on it, but it doesn't serve you, your family or your health, which means it's time to Let It GO! So here it is... BOTTOM LINE, either throw all the bad stuff out or donate it, but you need to remove it from the house IMMEDIATELY. If you merely put them to the side, you or a family member will be apt to put them back and you will find them again next year. Make your life easy, just get rid of it!

Family SuperPower Food List

Shopping List	Substitutions

Favorite Foods	Substitutions

Next up...PREPARATION for Success!!

Life has so many challenges that arise on a day-to-day basis. Creating a healthy kitchen needs good weekly preparation to make the everyday routine move along with ease. Just as with any goal a good plan is what creates success and will make the work of preparing healthy meals that much easier. The key here is to create a plan that involves the family. I realize that you may be thinking that this will be near to impossible, but remember that every moment of involvement that you create for the family is a learning lesson for life. Get everyone involved, let them choose their jobs or pull them out of a hat, either way these are amazing lessons that will help through college and beyond. You know your family best; create the right motivation and cheer them on, these challenges and lessons will shine bright as they become adults.

We all have different ways of doing things, for ease and comfort try to do what you think works best for your family. In my experience and with my own family we practice "Meal Prep Sundays". Choose the day that works for you and then divide the workload among your crew.

Meal Prep Made Simple:

- ♣ Pick a day of the week when you will set the menu for the following week, get the family involved. Choose at least one new recipe per week (or per month, let's face it life does get crazy).

♣ Review your current inventory and make a list of all the ingredients that you need to buy. Here's a good place to motivate an older sibling to create a master shopping spreadsheet, just a thought.

♣ Pick a day for your grocery shopping (or, if you want to have more time, sign up for a service that will deliver them to your door).

♣ Pick a day for food prep, preferably a weekend when the entire family can help. This is the day you will measure, cook, and store your foods in containers and/or ziplock type bags for the days ahead. This is a great time for the little ones to decide and organize their daily snacks for school, etc.

It is interesting to see how nowadays we eat out strictly out of convenience. Eating at home has become a chore, but I would like to encourage you to change that. Change can have its challenges, but once you set up your systems in place, this should all become part of the day-to-day life in your home and it should be easy!

Everything you have learned so far was given to you to make your kitchen healthier and meals easier, NOT to stress you out any more than need be. Most of us are pretty busy in our day-to-day lives; whether you are a mom, student or working full time, it can be hard (or you may think absolutely impossible!) to cook all of your meals at home each day. This is where meal preparation (aka "meal prep") can quickly become your best friend! Without meal prep, you increase your chances of eating junk or convenience foods if you get busy or caught without food.

So what is meal prep? Meal prep can mean different things to different people, so it is important you find a routine that works for you. Essentially, it should save you time in the kitchen and make it easier for you to eat healthier during the week.

How to Meal Prep

The first thing you need to do is invest in some good quality airtight containers, these can be BPA-free plastic or the glass variety. I suggest using glass for the home and choosing either stainless steel or BPA-free plastic for "on the go" meals and snacks. Keep in mind that if you are going to be reheating your food in these you want to choose ones that are oven safe. It is a good idea to buy containers that are the same sizes so they can be easily stacked in your fridge.

Best products for easy meal prep:

Here are my top 10, made easy, kitchen "must-haves":

- ✓ Food Containers – Ensure they are airtight & BPA-free!
- ✓ Mini Waffle Maker – Great for protein pancakes
- ✓ High Speed Blender – For healthy smoothies
- ✓ Knives, Scissors, and Sharpener – Sharp for chopping veggies
- ✓ Measuring Cups & Spoons – Ensure portions for recipes
- ✓ Food Saver – Great airtight packaging for freezing and storing
- ✓ Insulated Lunch Bag – For lunches on the go
- ✓ Reusable Ziploc Storage Bags – Gallon size
- ✓ Reusable Snack bags – Awesome for raw nuts & snacks
- ✓ Sharpies and Dry erase markers – To mark on containers and food packages

How to get started:

1. Check your calendar – what do you have going on this week?
2. Decide on the recipes for the week
3. Take a look in your pantry – what do you already have that you can use?
4. Make a shopping list of everything you need
5. After shopping, sort foods on the counter into "make now" and "make later" piles.

Once you get home from the store:

1. Wash and prep fruit and vegetables. Cut them up, store in containers or baggies in the fridge.
2. Bake or grill your chicken and brown your meat or simply store it marinated to be cooked. I shred or cube cooked chicken and store it in a large container in the fridge to use throughout the week. You could divide it into each container for the day to be used. As a general rule, your cooked meat will last for 3–4 days in the refrigerator. (And for those days or weeks when life has you on the run buy an organic cooked chicken and make your life easy.)
3. Cook quinoa & oats and store in containers. As a general rule, most grains will last for 3–5 days when cooked plain. Also take note of some of the Overnight Oat recipes I have here in this book, you can set up 3 days' worth of jars with the fruit and liquid and an additional 3 days with only the dry goods.
4. And then label everything. You can use dry erase markers on plastic containers or sharpies on plastic bags. If you want to get really organized and creative, you can have a different color for each day of the week.

Meal Prep Tip #1: *Make foods accessible*

Make your healthy foods look organized and beautiful in your fridge! Keep your healthy foods in airtight containers. Then, when those cravings set in, it's easy to grab something good for you, and you are less likely to feel the need to go "grab something fast" from the store. This is the best situation for your kids as well, make things like carrot and celery sticks easy to grab on the lower shelves. Have hummus or some other favorite bean dip available to dip into. The easier it is to see and grab the more often they will reach for these healthier alternatives. Plus, the fact that they assisted in choosing, making, and organizing helps as well.

Meal Prep Tip #2: *Keep the junk OUT*

Don't even bring the junk into your house PERIOD! We all know that our kids will eat junk at other people's houses, so keep your house as a healthy sanctuary. "Out of Sight, Out of Mind," and then for those rare occasions when you need chips or such for a gathering—HIDE THEM! Let's not instill any habits of mindless grazing on JUNK; we are here to teach our children to feed their bodies with nutrients for growth and development

Meal Prep Tip #3: *Use your freezer to store backups*

Your freezer is your backup reserve! Here is the place where you store your animal proteins, "smooshy" fruit for smoothies (you know the ones, the fruit that the kids refuse to eat because it got soft or changed color but is still good – freeze this stuff for smoothies!), veggies, nuts, and more. Typically, when the refrigerator runs out, the freezer kicks in!

You can't make this stuff up...

Backstory — I have been hiding ingredients in my kids' food since birth (or around then, you know what I mean).

Until the age of 5, if you asked my daughter if she liked garlic, onions, or even tomatoes she would give you a definitive NO, no way, no how!

Around that age I encouraged her to help me more and more in the kitchen and told her that she had been eating most of those ingredients since birth. One of her favorite meals is a ground beef picadillo with rice or quinoa. Her version is plain meat with rice, or at least that is what she thought it was until I had her blend up the "seasoning"...garlic, onions, tomatoes, peppers, and kale.

Now when someone asks if she likes Garlic she replies, "Yup I guess I do and I always have".

Notes, Stuff to Remember, Things to Buy, etc.

Family Friendly Recipes

The key to preparing the right foods for the family is to understand their basic pallet. Do they like sweet or salty? Meat, chicken or fish or do they prefer veggies? It's all good; every meal or snack should include a carbohydrate (preferably from fruits or veggies), a protein, and a bit of quality fat. A well-thought-out meal should be able to adapt to a variety of pallets without making separate meals for each. This section, although not a full cook book, will include some of my top recipes to get you started, but remember that, although a meal may be categorized as breakfast, you could easily eat it any time or for any meal—think outside of the box. One more thing; most of the recipes here are single serving so you can easily convert them for the number of people in your family. There are only a few that have a larger serving size, but those are marked!

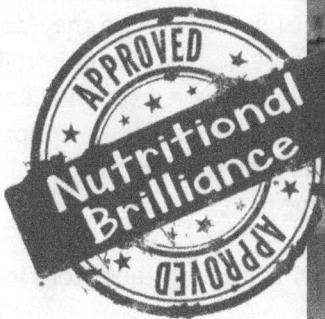

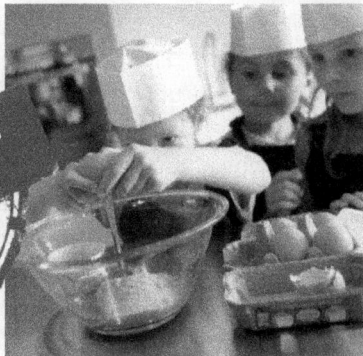

Breakfast

Breakfast (or snack) Muesli

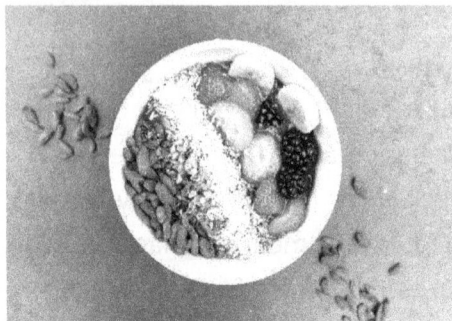

Here's a breakfast that will give you a good amount of quality protein, fats, and carbs for sustained energy and endurance throughout your day! Once combined, you can eat it with one of the great nut milks that are available. I like to set up a "bar" of sorts so that my family can spoon in each item the way they like it. I place each item in an airtight jar and leave them lined up on the counter.

What you will use:

Oats	Walnuts
Sliced Almonds	Dried Mulberries
Goji Berries	Coconut Flakes
Cinnamon	

Make it happen:

Mix in a big bowl and serve with nut milk. Get creative—you can mix just about any dried ingredient (just make sure they don't add any sugar or unidentifiable ingredients). There is rolled barley, rolled rye, raisins, etc. and you can even combine some fresh ones while you are serving it like berries or chopped apple. Just be sure to have ample protein ingredients, this is where your raw nuts and seeds come in.

Option: Make a big batch of the dry ingredients and store in an airtight jar for up to a month.

Quinoa Morning Eye Opener

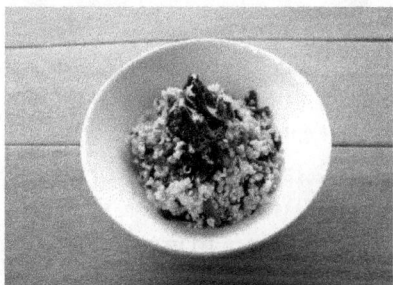

Quinoa is a great add-on to any meal; it is a complete protein and provides a whole array of amazing nutrients. My suggestion... Cook up a big batch plain then you can use it for so many different things throughout the week. As for breakfast, put a scoop of plain cooked quinoa into a cereal bowl, add in fresh cut fruit and berries and drizzle with a bit of honey.

Cacao Coco Delight Smoothie

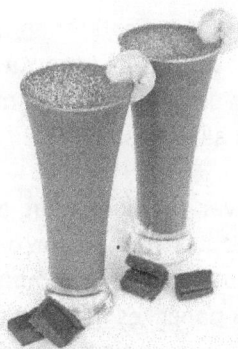

What you will use:
2 Cups of Coconut Milk
1 Banana
1 Teaspoon Cacao Nibs
6 Dates
2 Tablespoons Chia Seeds
1 Scoop of Vanilla Plant-Based Protein (or chocolate)
1 Teaspoon Vanilla
Pinch of Celtic Sea Salt

Make it happen:
Blend in a high speed blender until smooth and drink as a smoothie or freeze in fruit pops for a yummy treat.

Coconut Protein Pancakes

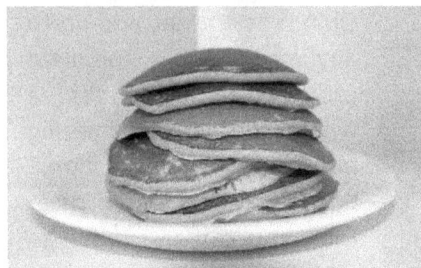

What you will use:
4 Eggs
1 Cup Coconut or Almond Milk
2 Tablespoons Coconut Oil (for the batter, then use extra to grease the skillet)
2 Tablespoons Honey or Maple Syrup
1/3 Cup Coconut Flour
1 Teaspoon Cinnamon
1 Teaspoon Vanilla
1/2 Teaspoon Baking Powder
1 Scoop of Vanilla Plant-Based Protein

Make it happen:
In a bowl whisk together all of the liquid ingredients, then add in the dry ingredients. You want the batter to be smooth so depending on what type of protein powder you use you may have to add a bit more of the milk. Whisk all until smooth.

Add some coconut oil to the skillet over medium heat and spoon mixture onto skillet. Cook for about 3 minutes or once bubbles start to form and then flip and cook for another minute or so. You will end up making approx. 15 pancakes and you can top them with either maple syrup or, my all-time favorite, pureed berries. *And if you want to make it even easier, use a waffle iron; yup, they come out like waffles and are super easy to make.

Option: Skip the maple syrup and simply puree some berries and pour that on top!

Overnight Oats

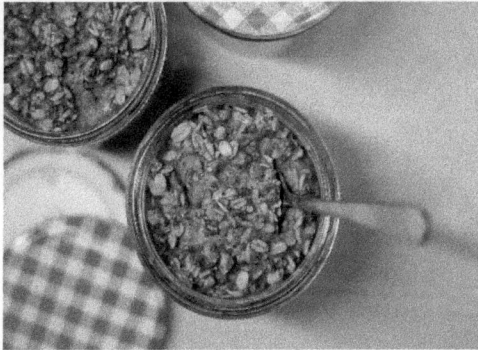

Here's the easiest way of packing in the nutrients into a "fast food", "grab when you need it" type package!

1. **Start with Rolled Oats.** Add these in with an equal amount of your liquid of choice. You can use any combination of almond, hemp or coconut milk; you can even use water, but be sure to add in a few more berries for flavor and sweetness. For this, rolled oats seem to work best, you can use steel cut oats, but you would need to add in more liquid and be prepared to do some extra chewing.

2. **Next Up, Add in Your Flavors.** Here is where you can use spices like cinnamon and vanilla, even shredded coconut makes it yummy. Also you could add in a scoop of protein powder to give it an extra boost. Pureed dates, honey or stevia and any combination of berries you would enjoy will sweeten it up nicely.

3. **Top it off and Eat up!** For your grand finale add in nut mix or sliced nuts and store in a glass jar or airtight container and let the oats soak for at least three hours, ideally overnight.

Option: If you want to create a few days' worth, then soak only the oats and add in the toppings as you're racing out the door. This works great with recycled almond butter jars.

Orange Vanilla Overnight Oats

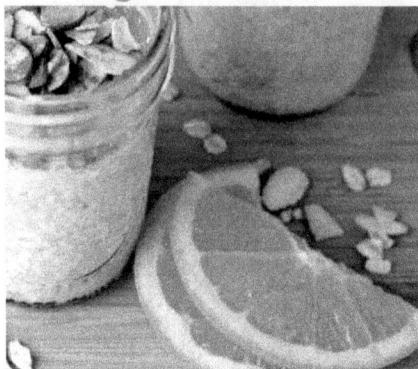

So very yummy! It's all the same as above but the oats are soaked in freshly squeezed orange juice. Then follow the layers, add in more vanilla as your spice of choice and layer in coconut flakes, nut mix, and fruit such as sliced mango and oranges. (You can easily add in a plant-based protein powder for an extra ounce of fuel!)

Maple Almond Butter Overnight Oats

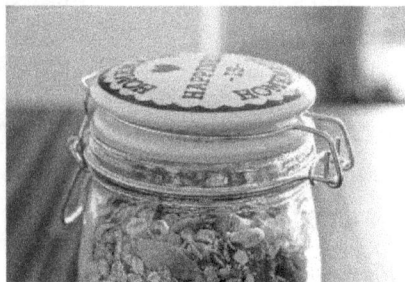

Start with your oats and almond milk.

Next layer comes about 1 tablespoon of chia seeds, some cinnamon, and a dash of vanilla.

Refrigerate and then, when you're about to serve, mix one banana with a heaped tablespoon of raw almond butter and add that to the oats. Top it off with a drizzle of maple syrup and a few pecans and you are set.

Snacks

Energy Bars

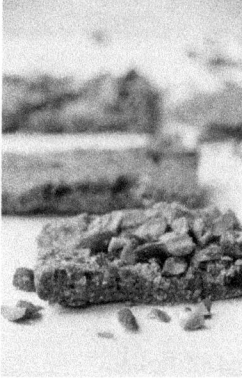

What you will use:

3 Cups Raw Pistachios
2 Cups Dried Mulberries
1 1/4 Cups Raw Cashew Butter
2/3 Cup Chia Seeds
1/4 Cup Honey
6 Dates
2 Teaspoons Vanilla
1 Teaspoon Cardamom
1 Teaspoon Cinnamon

Make it happen:

With the use of a food processor, start by finely chopping the pistachios, then put those to the side. Next chop the mulberries and dates, add in the cashew butter, chia seeds, honey, and spices. Take a pan with a one-inch edge, line it with wax paper and spread half of the chopped pistachios along the bottom of the pan. Spread the mulberry mixture on top of that and top that off with the remaining pistachios. Place in the refrigerator for about one hour then chop into squares and save in an airtight container and enjoy!

Zucchini Muffins, *Gluten Free!*

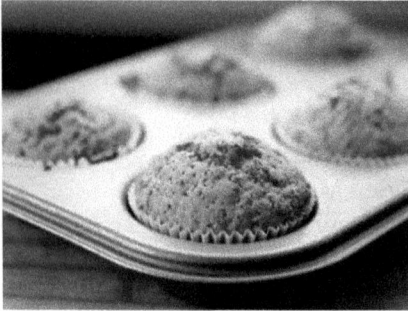

What you will use:
3 Cups Grated
Fresh Zucchini
1/2 Cup Coconut Oil
11 Medjool Dates
(blended with water until
smooth)
2 Teaspoons Maple Syrup
2 Eggs (beaten)
2 Teaspoons Vanilla
2 Teaspoons Baking Soda
Pinch of Celtic Sea Salt
3 Cups Flour (1/2 Cup Coconut and 2 1/2 Cups Oat flour)
2 Teaspoons Cinnamon
1/2 Teaspoons Nutmeg
1/2 Cup Adita's Nut Mix (this is optional but adds good quality
protein and fat, you can find the recipe at www.AditaLang.com)
1 Cup Mulberries (soaked in water until soft)

Make it happen:
1. Preheat oven to 350 degrees. In a large bowl combine the pureed dates, maple syrup, eggs, and vanilla. Stir in the grated zucchini and the coconut oil. In a separate bowl, mix the flour, baking soda, nutmeg, and cinnamon. Stir everything in together and add in mulberries.
2. Coat muffin or bread pan with olive oil and fill the cups up completely with batter. Bake on middle rack until golden brown and poke with a toothpick to make sure the inside is dry. Once cooked, remove from oven and let cool for about five minutes before removing from muffin or bread pans. After you have removed them from the pans, let cool for another 20 minutes.

Fruit Pops

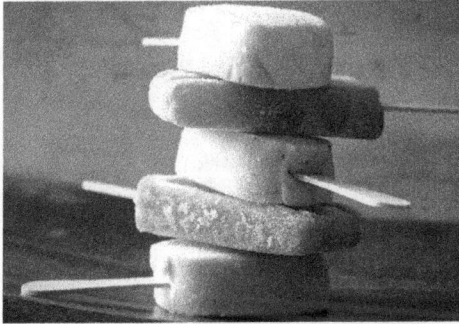

This is a fun-filled wild card. Remember your kids will love them if they are sweet, but the goal is to do this without added sugar and to include an adequate amount of protein.

What you will use;

First let's start with the liquid – Coconut Water, Coconut Milk, Plain Water, Hemp Milk, and Almond Milk.

Here's what makes them **SWEET** – Dates, Pears, Bananas, Watermelon, Mango, and any other sweet fruit in season.
Here's what makes them **POWERFUL** – Goji Berries, Spinach, Kale, Collard Greens, Avocado, Coconut.

Here's what gives it **PROTEIN** – Hemp Seeds, Raw Almond Butter, Raw Cashew Butter or a Plant-Based Protein Powder – kids like vanilla or chocolate best.

So here's what you do next; for you first-timers, start off by choosing a liquid that works for you and the kids. Next add in only fruit, make it tasty and blend it up in a high speed blender. Then add in a little bit of POWER and PROTEIN, blend it, taste it—if it's not sweet enough add in more fruit and Make it Tasty! Then freeze it in Popsicle sleeves or ice cube containers with toothpicks as handles. Now here's the trick, each time you make them add in more POWER and PROTEIN, your goal is to have an even mix of everything in a tasty treat that your family loves. My kids will eat several in a day and I love it—I know they are getting so much nutrition that I couldn't be happier. And better yet, these are my favorites after a good workout on a hot day!

Hummus Pizza

What you will use:

1 Cup of Garbanzos
1 Clove of Garlic
1Teaspoon of Tahini
1 1/2 Tablespoons of Hemp Seeds
A dash of Celtic Sea Salt
1 Tablespoon of Water
Olive Oil
Ezekiel Wraps

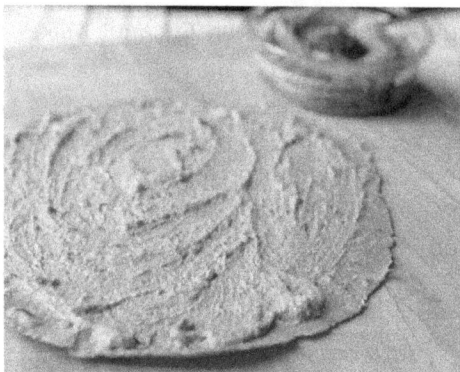

Make it happen:

Place the garlic in a high speed blender or food processor; next add in the hemp seeds, then add in the garbanzos, tahini, Celtic sea salt and 2 T of olive oil. Gradually add in more olive oil or water as a means of creating smoothness. Once the hummus is ready, spread it evenly on an Ezekiel wrap and cover with another wrap. Heat up a pan with some olive oil and place the "pizza" in the pan and lightly brown on both sides. Cut into diagonal slices and enjoy. You can also add in a bit of cheese or sundried tomatoes inside with the hummus.

Ants in a Log

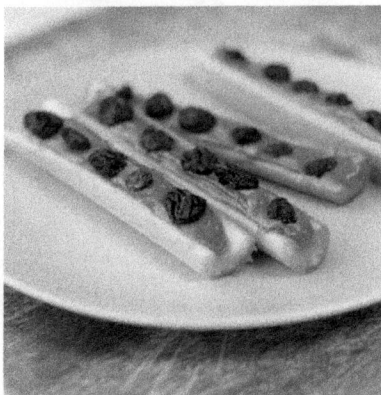

Make it happen:
Cut pieces of Celery into two-inch pieces.

In a bowl combine your favorite Raw Nut Butters (almond, cashew, pecan, etc.) with my Nut Mix.

Fill the Celery crevasse with your Nut Butter Mix.

Then top then with a row of your favorite Organic Dried or Fresh Berries (raisins, mulberries, golden berries, goji berries, blue berries, etc.).

Creamsicle Smoothie

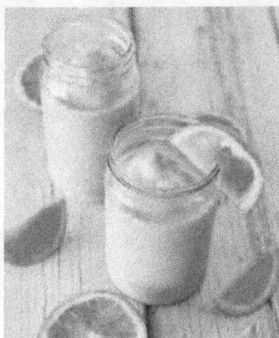

What you will use:
1 Cup Hemp, Almond or Coconut Milk
1 Teaspoon Vanilla
1/2 Cup freshly squeezed Orange Juice
1 Teaspoon Orange Zest (simply grate the rind of the orange)
1 Scoop of Vanilla Plant-Based Protein
5 Dates
1 Cup of Ice
2 Teaspoons of Adita's Nut Mix

Make it happen:
Blend everything together in a high speed blender and enjoy!
*Note - This makes an amazing frozen fruit pop.

Mango Mint Smoothie

What you will use:

1 Cup Hemp, Almond or Coconut Milk
1 Teaspoon Vanilla
1/2 Cup freshly squeezed Orange Juice
1 Teaspoon Orange Zest (simply grade the rind of the orange)
1 Scoop of Vanilla Protein Powder (I recommend Vanilla Superfoods Mix)
5 Dates
1 Cup of Ice
2 Teaspoons of Adita's Nut Mix

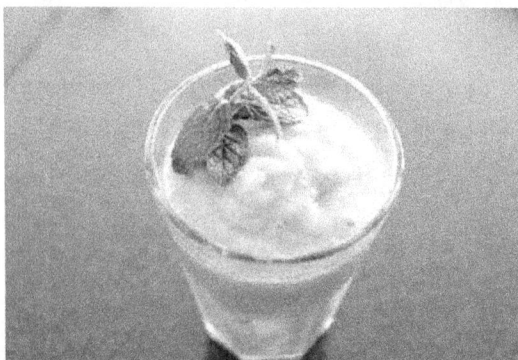

Make it happen:

Blend everything together in a high speed blender and enjoy!
*Note - This makes an amazing frozen fruit pop.

Kale Chips

What you will use:
3 Stalks Organic Kale, stalk removed and roughly chopped
1 Tablespoon Olive Oil
Celtic Sea Salt, to taste

Make it happen:
Preheat oven to 250 degrees, toss Kale with olive oil in a large bowl. Arrange all in a single layer on a non-stick baking sheet and sprinkle with sea salt. Bake for 30 to 33 minutes, watching closely not to overcook—you want them crispy. Allow to cool before serving.

Lunch

Nut Butter and Honey Sandwich:

What you will use:

Ezekiel Bread or Wrap
Organic Raw Nut Butter (almond, cashew, pecan, etc.)
Honey or a Mashed-Up Banana (for an extra immune booster use Manuka Honey)
Adita's Nut Mix

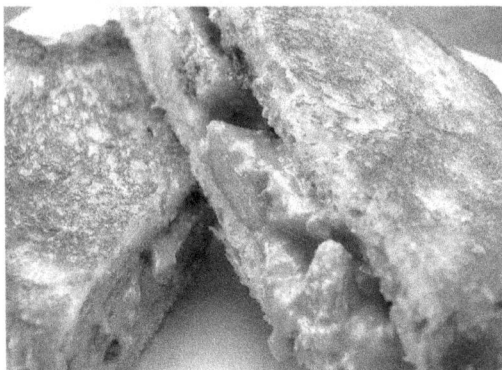

Make it happen:

Blend all ingredients together and spread on as a sandwich or wrap. Who said anyone needs to settle for a boring P&J sandwich? This one carries a nutritional punch and is just as yummy.

Egg and Avocado Wrap

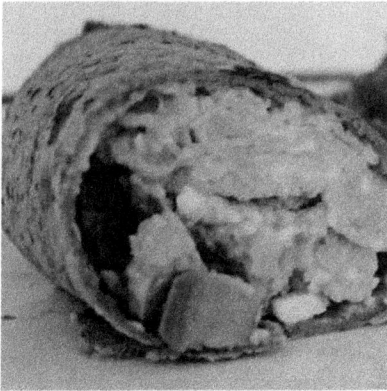

What you will use:

A wrap is a great way to make a meal on the go.

Eggs (any way you like them)
Sliced Avocado
Hemp Seeds
Ezekiel Wrap
Fresh Salsa

Make it happen:

Go ahead and get crazy—add in other veggies, a drizzle of olive oil, and a pinch of salt.

Chicken Salad Wrap

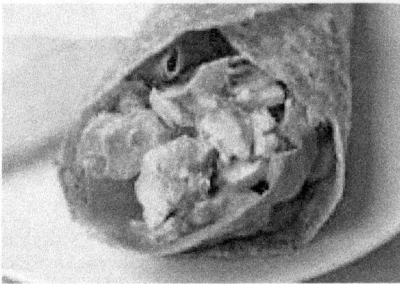

What you will use:

Cooked Organic Chicken
Avocado
Celtic Sea Salt
Olive Oil
Ezekiel Wrap

Make it happen:

Shred the chicken and combine it with mashed avocado. Next, place inside an Ezekiel wrap and drizzle olive oil and a dash of Celtic sea salt to taste. For an added nutritional boost, without changing the flavor, add in some hemp seeds.

143

Cauliflower Tabbouleh

What you will use:

1 large Cauliflower
1 Cup Fresh Parsley
1 1/2 Cups Chopped Cherry Tomatoes
1/2 Cup Cilantro
1/4 Cup Fresh Mint
1 Medium-Chopped Cucumber
1 Large Garlic Clove finely chopped

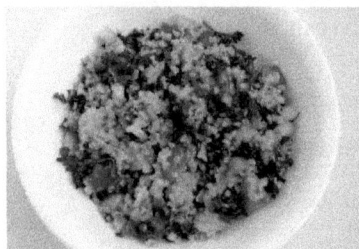

1/2 Cup Raw Chopped Almonds
1/2 Cup Lemon Juice
Olive Oil to taste
Celtic Sea Salt to taste
Optional: For added protein add in Hemp Seeds and Garbanzo Beans

Make it happen:

Chop cauliflower florets and place them into a food processor—chop until they reach rice like consistency. Place into a large bowl and combine the rest of the ingredients. Mix well and serve. **SERVES 5**

Garbanzo Bean Salad

What you will use:
1 Cup Garbanzo Beans, rinsed and drained (canned is fine – look for low salt)
1 Cup Cubed (1/2 inch) Cucumber
2 Cup Cubed (1/2 inch) Tomato
1 Cup Cubed (1/2 inch) Sweet Yellow Onion
2 Tablespoons Red Wine Vinegar
1 Tablespoon Extra Virgin Olive Oil
2 Tablespoons Finely-Chopped Basil or Mint

1 Tablespoon Finely-Chopped Parsley
Salt and Pepper to taste

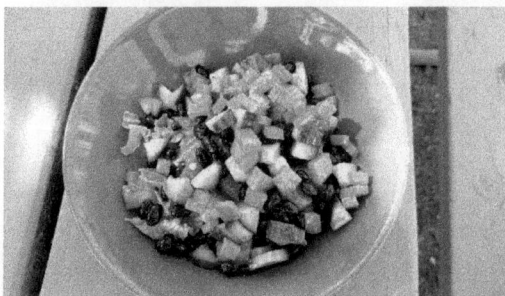

Make it happen:
Mix all together and let stand for a 1/2 hour. Serve on a bed of quinoa. This recipe will stay well in the refrigerator for up to 4 days – store salad and quinoa separately. **SERVES 6**

Zucchini Pizza

What you will use:

4 Large Zucchini
2 Finley-Chopped Large Tomatoes
5 Finley-Chopped Sun-Dried Tomatoes
1/2 Tablespoon Fresh Garlic

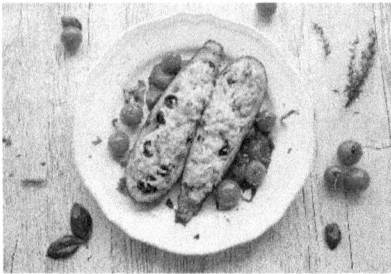

1/4 Teaspoon Oregano
1/4 Teaspoon Dried Basil or
12 Large Fresh Basil Leaves
Salt to taste
 *For the Cheese Lovers -
Grated Fresh
Parmigiano Cheese

Make it happen::

On the stove top sauté the garlic, tomatoes, sun-dried tomatoes, oregano, and dried basil (if you opt for fresh leaves leave these for right before putting on the cheese). Sauté for a couple of minutes.

Cut the Zucchini in half lengthwise, place in a roasting pan with the cut side up. Spread the tops with the sautéed mixture and add the cheese (they can be made with or without cheese). Place in the oven at 350 for about 35 minutes and enjoy!

Mexican Pizza

What you will use:

1 Ezekiel 4:9 Sprouted Grain Tortilla
3 oz. Organic Oven Roasted Chicken Breast, skinless
1/4 Cup Mild Salsa, if you like it hotter, go for it
1/2 Cup Red Peppers, chopped
2 Tablespoons Green Chili Peppers, diced
1 Cup Spinach
2 Tablespoons Organic Mozzarella Cheese, shredded (you can easily substitute with hummus)

1/4 Cup Avocado, sliced
1 Tablespoon Olive Oil

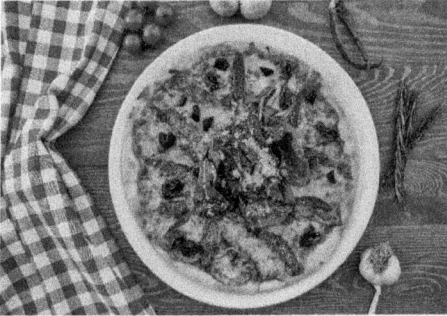

Make it happen:

Preheat oven to 450 degrees and lightly rub pan with olive oil. On the stove top cook bell peppers, green chilies and spinach on medium heat until spinach is wilted. Spread salsa on tortilla with chicken and spinach mixture. Sprinkle with cheese and bake until cheese melts. Top with avocado slices.

Dinner

Turkey and Bean Chili

What you will use:

1 Tablespoon Olive Oil
2 Garlic Cloves, minced
1 lb. Hormone and
Antibiotic-Free Ground
Turkey
2 Cans Low-Sodium Organic
Black Beans or Cannellini
Beans, drained and rinsed
1 Can Tomato Sauce
1 Tablespoon Chili Powder
1 Cup Onions, chopped
1 Green Bell Pepper, diced
1 Can Diced Tomatoes with Green Chilies
1 Cup Organic Corn, fresh or frozen

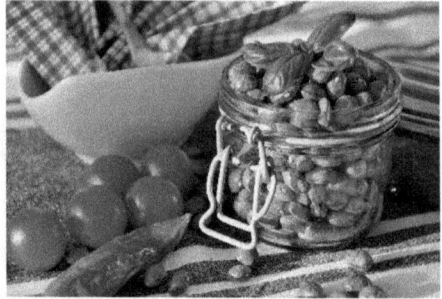

Make it happen:

In a soup pot or crock pot, heat the olive oil over a medium heat. Add the onions, garlic and bell pepper. Sauté for about three minutes or until slightly softened. Add turkey and sauté for another 6–7 minutes or until no longer pink, crumbling the meat with a spoon as it cooks. Add the beans, tomatoes, tomato sauce, corn, chili powder, and oregano. Bring to a boil, reduce the heat, and simmer for 15 minutes. (This recipe provides 4 servings. You can freeze the additional servings easily or keep them in an airtight container in the refrigerator for up to 4 days.) **SERVES 4**

Barbecue Chicken and Black Bean Burrito

What you will use:

1 Tablespoon Olive Oil
3 oz. Skinless, Boneless Organic Chicken Breast, cut into bite-size pieces (5 oz. for men)
2 Slices of Onion, finely chopped
1 Clove of Garlic, minced

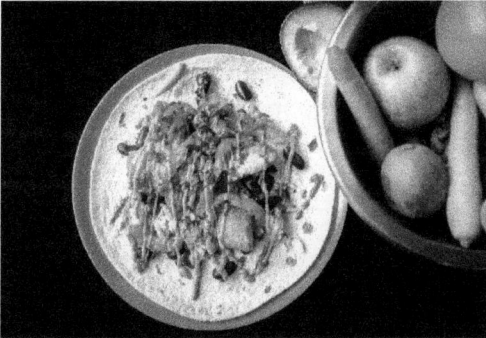

2 Tablespoons Organic Barbecue Sauce
1/2 Cup Organic Black Beans, rinsed and drained
2 Ezekiel 4:9 Sprouted Grain Tortillas

Make it happen:

Heat olive oil in a large skillet over medium heat; add chicken, onion and garlic. Cook for 8 minutes or until chicken is fully cooked, stirring constantly. Stir in barbecue sauce and beans; cook 5 more minutes or until thoroughly heated. Warm tortillas in a skillet until lightly browned. Divide the chicken mixture for each tortilla down the center of the tortilla and roll up.

Mahi Mahi Tacos

What you will use:

1 Tablespoon Fresh Lime Juice
1 Tablespoon Fresh Orange Juice
1 Garlic Clove, chopped
1/2 Teaspoon Chili Powder
Celtic Sea Salt and Pepper, to taste
A Dash of Cayenne Pepper
3 oz. of Wild Mahi Mahi, cut into bite-sized chunks (5 oz. for men)
1/2 of a Large Ripe Mango, peeled, pitted and chopped
2 Tablespoons Fresh Cilantro Leaves, chopped
1/8 Teaspoon Red Chili, seeded and chopped
2 Teaspoons Coconut Oil
2 Ezekiel 4:9 Sprouted Grain Tortilla
1/2 Ripe Tomato, peeled and chopped

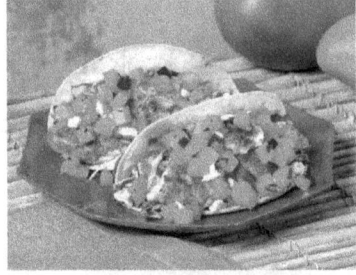

Make it happen:

In a medium bowl whisk together 1/2 tablespoon of lime juice, 1/2 tablespoon of orange juice, garlic, chili powder, salt, pepper, and cayenne pepper. Add the fish and gently stir to coat. Let stand for at least 10 minutes.

In a medium bowl combine the mango, onion, cilantro, chili and remaining lime and orange juice. Stir gently until well combined. Set aside in the refrigerator if you are marinating the fish longer than a few minutes. Let stand at room temperature for at least 20 minutes before serving. In a large cast iron skillet, heat the olive oil over medium heat. Add the fish and its marinade and cook for 3 to 4 minutes turning frequently until the fish is opaque. While the fish cooks, heat the tortilla on a skillet until light brown. Gently fold the avocado into the mango mixture. Divide all of the ingredients into both tortillas and enjoy!

Roasted POWER Brussel Sprouts

What you will use:

10 Brussels Sprouts, chopped into quarters
1/2 Cup Quinoa
1/2 Cup Cannellini Beans
2 Tablespoons Olive Oil
1/2 Tablespoon Balsamic Vinegar
1 Tablespoon Organic Maple Syrup

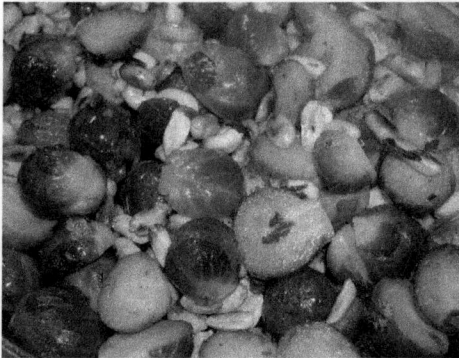

1 Cup Kale, chopped
2 Tablespoons Sun-Dried Tomatoes, finely chopped
1 Clove of Garlic, minced
Black Pepper, to taste
Celtic Sea Salt, to taste

Make it happen:

Rinse the quinoa and place in a pot with the water. Bring to a boil and cover, reduce the heat and cook until the water is absorbed, about 10–15 minutes. While the quinoa is cooking, take a deep baking dish and place the Brussels sprouts, olive oil, vinegar, maple syrup, garlic, pepper and salt and mix. Bake at 400 degrees for 25 minutes. Next, take out the Brussels sprouts and add in the beans and sun-dried tomatoes and mix well with the Brussels sprouts; return to the oven for 10 minutes or until the Brussels sprouts are crispy. Layer the quinoa, kale, and Brussels sprouts on a plate and enjoy!

Dessert

Raw Chocolate Pudding

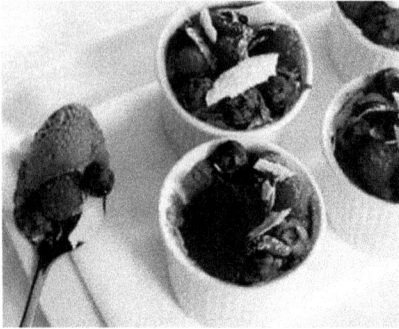

What you will use:
1 Cup Chia Seeds
1 1/2 Cups Coconut Milk
2 Tablespoons Raw Cacao
Powder
2 Tablespoons Pureed
Dates
1 Tablespoon Honey

Make it happen:
Mix all of the ingredients and place in the refrigerator to cool. The chia seeds will end up absorbing all of the liquid; once absorbed, place into a high speed blender and blend until smooth. You may need to add a bit of water to improve the quality of the smoothness—do it gradually until desired smoothness is accomplished. * For a protein boost and some extra chocolate, add in a hefty scoop of a chocolate plant-based protein powder, and ... for extra sweetness puree some berries and mix it in with a swirl!

No-Bake Almond Cookies

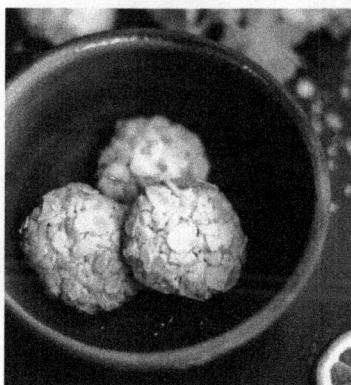

What you will use:
1 Cup Raw Almonds
1 Cup (about 10) Medjool Dates, pitted & chopped
1/2 Cup Almond Butter
1 1/2 Tablespoons Cacaos Nibs (optional)
2 Teaspoons Vanilla Extract
1/4 Teaspoon Celtic Sea Salt

Make it happen:
Place the almonds in a food processor or a mini chopper and pulse until it resembles a coarse meal. Add the dates, almond butter, vanilla, and salt. Pulse for a couple minutes until it forms a dough. Stir in cacao nibs, if using. You can use your hands to knead in the cacao nibs as the dough is thick.

Shape about one tablespoon of dough into a round cookie shape and place on parchment paper. Enjoy right away or place the cookies into the fridge for storage.

No-Bake Vegan Brownies

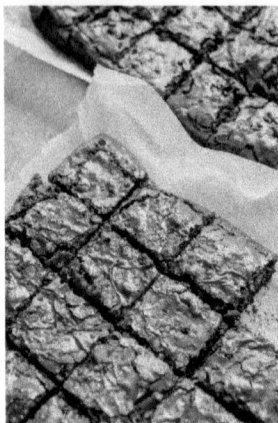

What you will use:
2 Cups Rolled Oats
1 Cup Raw Cashews
8 Dates, pitted
1/3 Cup Raw Cocoa Powder
1/4 Teaspoon Celtic Sea Salt
1 Ripe Banana
1/4 Cup Applesauce
1/4 Cup Chopped Walnuts

Make it happen:
Place the oats, cashews, dates, cocoa powder, and salt in a food processor and blend until everything is a smooth, floury consistency. Add the banana and applesauce and blend until a thick, slightly sticky dough forms.

Lightly grease (with coconut oil) a 7x11 pan. Push the mixture into the pan firmly using the back of a spatula. Top with chopped walnuts, pushing them into the dough. Place pan in the fridge for at least an hour to firm up. Cut into 32 squares, and store uneaten brownies in the fridge.

Chocolate Coconut Balls

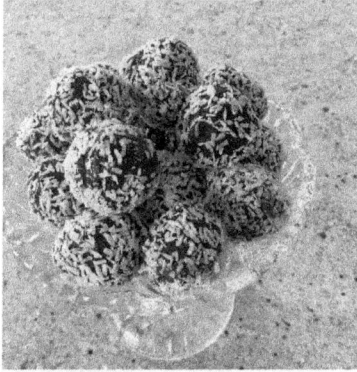

What you will use:
2 Cups Dates
1 Cup Raw Cashews
1/2 Cup Raw Sunflower Seeds
1/4 Cup Unsweetened
Shredded Coconut
1 Scoop Plant-Based Protein
Powder (either vanilla or
chocolate)
1/4 Cup Raw Powdered Cacao
2 Tablespoons Coconut Oil

2 Tablespoons Honey
1 Teaspoon Cinnamon

Make it happen:
In a food processor finely chop the dates, cashews, and sunflower seeds. Next add in the rest of the ingredients and blend up until you have a smooth doughy texture. Roll into a one-inch ball and then roll onto additional shredded coconut for an outer coating. Place on a cookie sheet covered with wax paper and let set in refrigerator for about an hour. Store in an airtight container and enjoy!

Receive my latest recipes right in your inbox, sign up at www.AditaLang.com

Sweet Longevity Chocolate Mousse

What you will use:
3/4 Cup Dates, soaked until very soft with pits removed
1 Tablespoon Coconut Butter
1 Cup Almond Milk
1/2 Cup Almond Butter
3/4 Cup Cacao Powder
1 Tablespoon Honey
Fresh Raspberries to top with

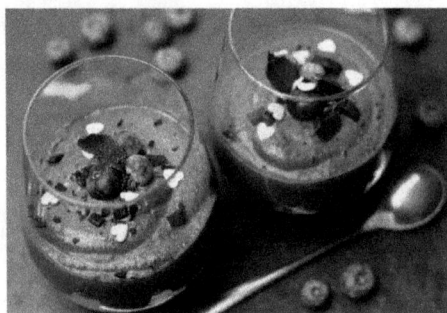

Make it happen:
In a high speed blender, combine all ingredients and blend until smooth. Refrigerate, and then enjoy your sweets with pure delight! Oh, one more thing... You can puree berries as a drizzly topping or just add them whole for some extra sweetness.

Here is one Yummy Idea:
Cupcakes! Line 16 mini muffin cups with cupcake paper liners. Spoon a small scoop of mousse into each paper liner. Place the muffin tin in the freezer for at least 30 minutes to harden. Remove from freezer, top with a raspberry and now you have a cupcake! Yummy!

Ultimate Longevity Food Substitution List

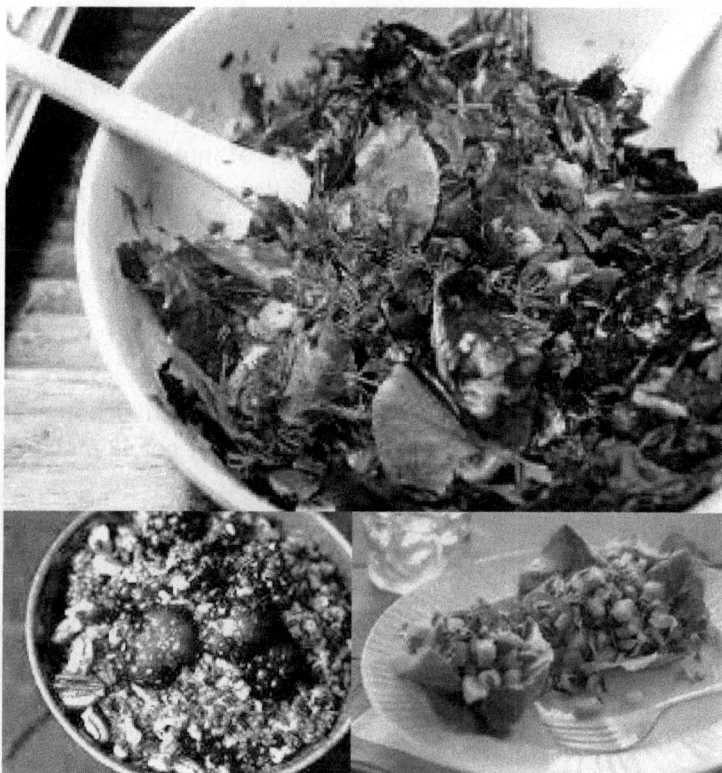

Ideas for Main Meals

Avocado mash for mayo

Mayonnaise has about 200 plus calories, while the same serving of avocado only brings in about half of that with an array of essential vitamins and minerals ... hmmm. So without giving it a thought, smash up an avocado and add it anyplace you would use mayo!

Arugula, romaine, spinach, collards and kale for iceberg lettuce

Darker green leaves are packed full of nutrients like iron, vitamin C, and antioxidants. The pale leaves of iceberg lettuce have no chance to even compare. Make each bite count and go for the nutrient-dense varieties!

Coconut milk for cream

Coconut milk is a great exchange for heavy cream in soups and stews. It may bring a bit of coconut flavor but not so much that you can't cover it up with spices and more.

Lettuce leaves for tortilla wraps

Any wrap dish or taco can be replaced with a large lettuce or greens leaf! Here's a great way to lower the processed carbs and enhance the nutrition.

Nuts for croutons (in salads)

Have you seen my famous Nut Mix? Yup, it's an ideal way of adding protein and quality fat to a salad without the carbs and additives that croutons bring. Take an array of raw nuts and seeds and blend them to a coarse powder and have at it! Check out my video at http://youtu.be/9W9IGbd2qp0

Pureed fruit for syrup

Syrup for pancakes and syrup for waffles… Who needs syrup when you can take some fresh berries and puree them up for a sweet delight?

Quinoa for oatmeal

You can easily cook quinoa with water or any nut milk; then add in mashed-up berries and you have a great protein-filled breakfast.

Quinoa for couscous

Couscous is made from processed wheat flour; quinoa is a whole-grain superfood packed with protein and nutrients. They have the same texture but one gives you so much more nutrition per bite!

Rolled oats for breadcrumbs

As I always say, "Minimize the Gluten!" Traditional breadcrumbs are filled with all sorts of additives and more; on the other hand, rolled oats can be seasoned up with herbs to make an amazing breading alternative.

Spaghetti squash for pasta

Steamed in the oven and pulled apart with a fork, spaghetti squash is a great low-carb and lower-calorie substitute for pasta. One squash will make between two and three servings.

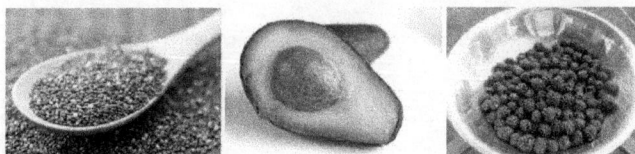

Ideas for Snack Items

Frozen Grapes for a summertime snack

Freeze grapes without the stems and pass out the bags for a great snack on a hot day. Who needs candy?

Frozen Smoothie for frozen ice pops

As long as they are sweet your kids will love them, so take full advantage. Add in greens like collard green or cilantro, and then sweeten with dates and bananas and add in other fruits in between. I even add in protein powder for that extra bonus. Find these on p.137

Kale chips for potato chips

Once you have gone kale, there is no turning back! Toss in olive oil and some seasonings of choice, then broil on low—but keep your eye on the prize as they only take a few minutes and can burn very easily. This will become your "go-to" crunch snack with less fat than any potato chip out there! Find these on p. 141

Ideas for Baking

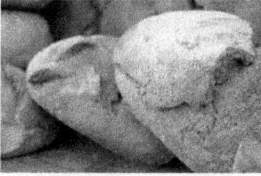

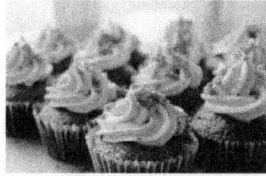

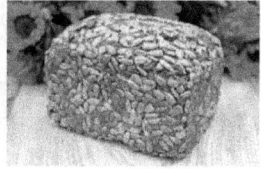

Almond flour / Nut flour for wheat flour

Too much gluten is not a good thing so here is a great way to up the protein and omega-3s in most of your baked goods! Keep in mind that the flavor is a bit nuttier than traditional flour and almond flour is much heavier, so when making your exchange think about using a 1/4 cup at the beginning (so 1 cup flour would become 3/4 cup flour and 1/4 cup almond flour). Or, if you want to take it full force and your recipe includes a rising agent, you may need to increase the amount of rising agent (by about 1/2 teaspoon per cup of almond flour added) to account for the extra weight. (**Nut flours do tend to be heavier than traditional flour, so make sure to up the amount of baking powder and baking soda in the recipe so the dough can rise as normal)

Avocado puree for butter (in anything chocolate!)

This is best done with any type of fudge or chocolate recipe so that the flavor of the avocado does not shine through. This exchange may take a few trial runs to get it right, but for the most part a 1:1 ratio works well.

Black beans for brownies!

Ditch the flour and add a can of black beans instead (drained and rinsed) in your favorite brownie recipe. This makes for a great way to pack in the protein and give a good kick to the gluten. When baking, exchange 1 cup of flour with 1 cup or a 15 oz. can of organic black beans and puree.

Cacao nibs for chocolate chips

The root of chocolate started out as... cacao nibs. This unprocessed alternative cuts out all of the additives, fat, and other stuff and leaves you with a nutrient-dense alternative. You have to play around with this one and make sure to sweeten it, but the sky's the limit as to what things you can make!

Chia seeds for eggs

It's more than your traditional Chia Pet. Combine 1 tablespoon chia seeds with 1 cup of water and let sit for 15 minutes to create a perfect 1:1 egg substitute for baking.

Coconut flour for flour

If you're looking at enhancing nutrients and removing some of the carbs from a baked treat, coconut flour works well as a partial exchange. Be careful though—using more than half a cup at a time could allow the flour's bitterness to take over. Your exchange can be tricky, so be sure to add an equal amount of extra liquid! For baking, you typically want to substitute only 1/4 to 1/3 cup of coconut flour for your 1 cup of traditional flour (so if it's 1/4 cup coconut flour, then you also have an additional 3/4 cup of your traditional flour).

Dates for sugar

It takes about 10 dates to exchange one cup of sugar, but this also gives you a bit of protein, tons of fiber, vitamin A, B, and K, folate, magnesium, phosphorus, potassium, and a lot more! So for the added nutrients and fiber this is a perfect exchange, the calories are about the same but the benefits are so much more!

Flax meal for eggs

Here's a vegan trick; mix 1 tablespoon of freshly ground flax seeds with 3 tablespoons of warm water and whisk well to combine. Next, let it sit in the refrigerator for 5–10 minutes before using as an exchange for 1 egg in any baked recipe.

Mashed bananas for fats

With a 1:1 ratio a perfectly soft and ripe banana can help the same as avocados to replace the fat in a baking recipe. The consistency works well and the nutritional punch adds in potassium, fiber, and vitamin B6.

Meringue for frosting

Typical frosting can add a good 300-plus calories to a basic cup cake, ugg! Meringue is made from egg whites and sugar; it's a great fat-free substitution for traditional frosting. Want to make it even cooler? Light a torch to it and that bit of charred delight will bring out the sweetness and caramelized flavor.

Unsweetened applesauce for baking

Using applesauce instead of sugar can give you all the sweetness with none of the added sugar, and that means fewer calories as well! One cup of applesauce contains only about 100 calories; a cup of sugar, on the other hand, can add in more than 700 calories! This exchange is ideal for cookies, muffins, and more. The exchange is a 1:1 ratio, but for every cup of applesauce, cut down on the amount of liquid in the recipe by 1/4 cup or so.

Want to eliminate the fat? Try applesauce instead of butter or oil in recipes like sweet bread, muffins, and more. Don't jump in full force at first, try exchanging only half the fat the first time around and see how that goes (so if you need 1 cup butter, try 1/2 cup applesauce and 1/2 cup butter). On the next round you'll know just how much works for your recipe.

Vanilla for sugar

Considering one cup of sugar can be about 800 calories, now think about cutting that in half and replacing it with vanilla extract. Now, it's a challenging exchange and may take a few trials on your part, but you can start by cutting 2 tablespoons of sugar and adding an extra 1/2 teaspoon of vanilla extract.

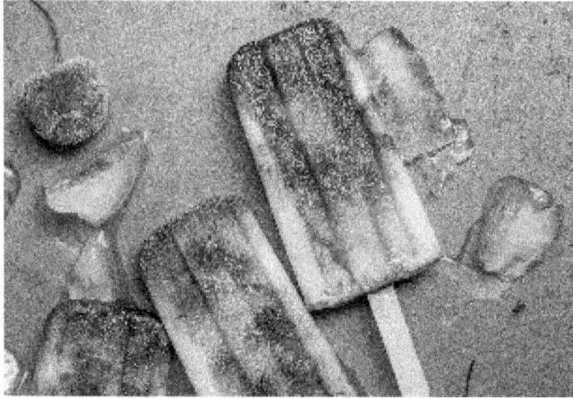

References

ACSM Issues New Recommendations on Quantity and Quality of Exercise. (2011, August 8). Retrieved from http://acsm.org/about-acsm/media-room/news-releases/2011/08/01/acsm-issues-new-recommendations-on-quantity-and-quality-of-exercise

Akerblom, H.K., et al., *Environmental factors in the etiology of type 1 diabetes. Am J Med Genet, 2002. 115(1): p. 18-29.*

American Academy of Family Physicians. (2003). *Eating Disorders: Facts for Teens.* Leawood, KS. Online and Custom Publishing-American Academy of Family Physicians. http://family doctor.org/277.xml

American Cancer Society 1701 Rickenbacker Drive Suite 5B Sun City Center, FL 33573-5361 (Educational material available) www.cancer.org

American College of Sports Medicine Position Stand. (2011). Retrieved from http://www.mhhe.com/hper/nutrition/williams/student/appendix_i.pdf

Appel, L.J., et al., *Effects of protein, monounsaturated fat, and carbohydrate intake on blood pressure and serum lipids:*

results of the OmniHeart randomized trial. *JAMA*, 2005. *294(19): p. 2455-64.*

Beachle, T. and R. Earle. (2004). *NSCA's Essentials of Personal Training*. Champaign, IL. Human Kinetics Publishers.

Bernardot, D. (1992). *Sports Nutrition-A Guide for the Professional Working with Active People*. 2nd Edition. Chicago, IL. American Dietetic Association.

Bernstein, A.M., et al., Dietary protein sources and the risk of stroke in men and women. Stroke, 2012. 43(3): p. 637-44.

Bernstein, A.M., et al., Major dietary protein sources and risk of coronary heart disease in women. Circulation, 2010. 122(9): p. 876-83.

Bonjour, J.P., Protein intake and bone health. Int J Vitam Nutr Res, 2011. 81(2-3): p. 134-42.

Chek, Paul. (2004). How to Eat, Move, and Be Healthy! San Diego, CA: A Chek Institute Publication.

Colgan, Dr. Michael. (1982). *Your Personal Vitamin Profile*. New York, NY. Quill

Darling, A.L., et al., Dietary protein and bone health: a systematic review and meta-analysis. Am J Clin Nutr, 2009. 90(6): p. 1674-92.

Deville, Nancy. (2007). *Death by Supermarket.* Ft. Lee, New Jersey: Barricade Books.

Dietary Guidelines Advisory Committee. (2005). *Dietary Guidelines for Americans*. Washington DC. U.S. Department of Health and Human Services and U.S. Department of Agriculture. www.healthierus.gov/dietaryguidelines

Escott-Stump S.*Nutrition and Diagnosis-Related Care*

Feskanich, D., et al., Protein consumption and bone fractures in women. Am J Epidemiol, 1996. 143(5): p. 472-9.

Food, Nutrition, Physical Activity, and the Prevention of Cancer: a Global Perspective. 2007, World Cancer Research Fund, American Institute for Cancer Research.: Washington, DC.

Halton, T.L., et al., Low-carbohydrate-diet score and the risk of coronary heart disease in women. N Engl J Med, 2006. 355(19): p. 1991-2002.

Institute of Medicine, Dietary Reference Intakes for Energy, Carbohydrate, Fiber, Fat, Fatty Acids, Cholesterol, Protein, and Amino Acids (Macronutrients). 2005, National Academies Press: Washington, DC.

Jenkins, D.J., et al., The effect of a plant-based low-carbohydrate ("Eco-Atkins") diet on body weight and blood lipid concentrations in hyperlipidemic subjects. Arch Intern Med, 2009. 169(11): p. 1046-54.

Kerstetter, J.E., A.M. Kenny, and K.L. Insogna, Dietary protein and skeletal health: a review of recent human research. Curr Opin Lipidol, 2011. 22(1): p. 16-20.

Kleiner S. (1999). Water: An Essential but Overlooked Nutrient. *Journal of the American Dietetic Association.* 99, pp. 200-206.

Lagiou, P., et al., Low carbohydrate-high protein diet and incidence of cardiovascular diseases in Swedish women: prospective cohort study. BMJ, 2012. 344: p. e4026.

Levey, Joel and Michelle. (1998). Living in Balance, Berkeley, CA: Conari Press.

Li SS, Kendall CW, de Souza RJ, Jayalath VH, Cozma AI, Ha V, Mirrahimi A, Chiavaroli L, Augustin LS, Blanco Mejia S, Leiter LA, Beyene J, Jenkins DJ, Sievenpiper JL. Dietary pulses, satiety and food intake: a systematic review and meta-analysis of acute feeding trials. Obesity, 2014. Aug;22(8):1773-80.

Mozaffarian, D., et al., Changes in diet and lifestyle and long-term weight gain in women and men. N Engl J Med, 2011. 364(25): p. 2392-404.

National Academy of Sciences. Institute of Medicine. Food and Nutrition Board. *Dietary Reference Intakes for Energy, Carbohydrate, Fiber, Fat, Fatty Acids, Cholesterol, Protein, and Amino Acids*

National Heart, Blood and Lung Institute. (2005). *High Blood Cholesterol, What You Need to Know.* Washington, DC. Department of Health and Human Services. NIH Publication No. 013290.

NIH Consensus Panel. (1993). Triglyceride, High Density Lipoprotein and Coronary Heart Disease. *Journal of the*

American Medical Association. Chicago, IL. 269, pp. 505-510.

Nutraterian Food Pyramid. (2011). Retrieved from www.EatRightAmerica.com

Oz, Mehmet and Roizen, Michael (2006). *You on a Diet*. New York, NY. Simon & Schuster, Inc.

Primack, Jeff. (2012). Conquering Any Disease. Press on Qi Prodctions.

Sleep – How to Maintain a Healthy Body Clock. (2012). Retrieved from http://www.fitness-n-function.co.nz/Wellness_Newsletter/Wake-Sleep.pdf

SMART Goals Template. (2012). Retrieved from http://www.hrg.stanford.edu/documents/SMARTGOALSTemplate2012.doc

SMART Goals. (2013). Retrieved from http://www.uwlax.edu/hr/current/idp/Smart%20Goal%20Worksheet.pdf

Sugar Science, University of California San Francisco www.SugarScience.org

The National Center for Nutrition and Dietetics, The American Dietetic Assoc. 215 West Jackson Blvd. Suite 800 Chicago, IL 1-800-366-1655 (Educational materials & referrals to dietitians) www.eatright.org

The National Diabetics education Initiative, Ashfield Healthcare Communications, Lyndhurst, NJ. http://www.ndei.org/index.aspx

United States Department of Agriculture. Center for Nutrition Policy and Promotion. *Dietary Guidelines for Americans. 2010.*

US Department of Agriculture Center for Nutrition Policy and Promotion 1120 20th ST. NW Suite 200, North Lobby Washington, DC 20036-3475 www.usda.com

US Department of Agriculture Center for Nutrition Policy and Promotion 1120 20th ST. NW Suite 200, North Lobby Washington, DC 20036-3475 www.usda.com

US Department of Health and Human Services Public Health Service National Heart, Lung, and Blood Institute www.hhs.gov

Wolcott, William and Fahey, Trish. (2000). *The Metabolic Typing Diet.* New York: Broadway Books.

Wolf, David. (2009). *Superfoods.* Berkeley, CA: North Atlantic Books.

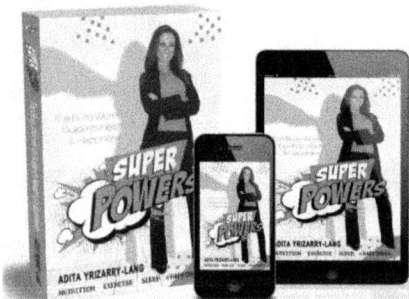

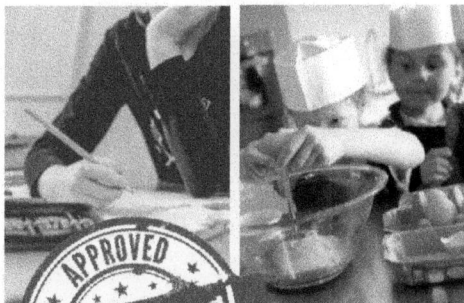

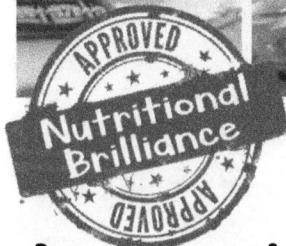

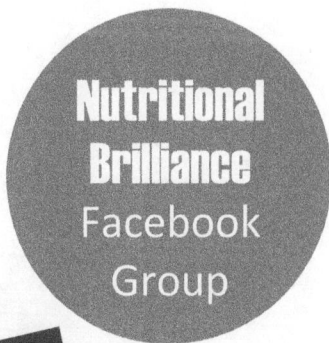

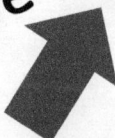

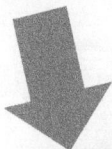

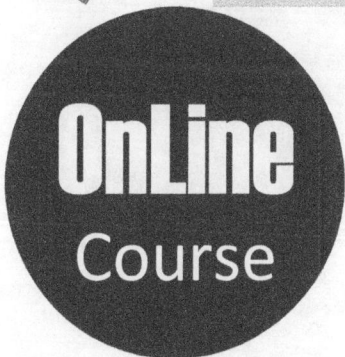

www.ingramcontent.com/pod-product-compliance
Lightning Source LLC
Chambersburg PA
CBHW060826050426
42453CB00008B/607